UNDERSTANDING INFECTIOUS DISEASES

The Deadliest Infectious Diseases

Andrea C. Nakaya

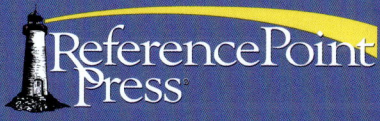

San Diego, CA

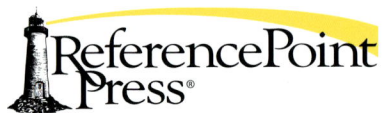

© 2022 ReferencePoint Press, Inc.
Printed in the United States

For more information, contact:
ReferencePoint Press, Inc.
PO Box 27779
San Diego, CA 92198
www.ReferencePointPress.com

ALL RIGHTS RESERVED.
No part of this work covered by the copyright hereon may be reproduced or used in any form or by any means—graphic, electronic, or mechanical, including photocopying, recording, taping, web distribution, or information storage retrieval systems—without the written permission of the publisher.

LIBRARY OF CONGRESS CATALOGING-IN-PUBLICATION DATA

Names: Nakaya, Andrea C., 1976- author.
Title: The deadliest infectious diseases / by Andrea C. Nakaya.
Description: San Diego, CA : ReferencePoint Press, [2022] | Series: Understanding infectious diseases | Includes bibliographical references and index.
Identifiers: LCCN 2021009641 (print) | LCCN 2021009642 (ebook) | ISBN 9781678201562 (library binding) | ISBN 9781678201579 (ebook)
Subjects: LCSH: Epidemics--Juvenile literature. | Communicable diseases--Juvenile literature.
Classification: LCC RA653.5 .N35 2022 (print) | LCC RA653.5 (ebook) | DDC 614.4--dc23
LC record available at https://lccn.loc.gov/2021009641
LC ebook record available at https://lccn.loc.gov/2021009642

CONTENTS

Introduction   4
    An Ongoing Threat

Chapter One   7
    About Infectious Diseases

Chapter Two   17
    Endemic Diseases

Chapter Three   26
    Epidemic and Pandemic Diseases

Chapter Four   36
    How Deadly Infectious Diseases Affect Society

Chapter Five   46
    Infectious Diseases in the Future

Source Notes   55
Organizations and Websites   58
For Further Research   59
Index   60
Picture Credits   64
About the Author   64

INTRODUCTION

An Ongoing Threat

In December 2019, cases of a mysterious, pneumonia-like illness began appearing in Wuhan, China. After a closer look, doctors discovered that this illness was caused by a new virus: a type of coronavirus that they named COVID-19. At first, health authorities simply monitored the situation. However, this cautious attitude soon gave way to widespread alarm as the new virus quickly began to spread and to kill. By the end of January 2020, numerous people had died from COVID-19, and cases had been reported in many other countries, including the United States.

More than a year later, COVID-19 had proven to be a deadly infectious disease, killing more than 2 million people worldwide, with no sign of stopping. In a December 2020 *Washington Post* article, Allison Wynes, a nurse in an intensive care unit in Iowa City, Iowa, talked about how the contagiousness and severity of this disease had overwhelmed the health care system. She compared fighting COVID-19 to controlling a raging fire. "I'm actually scared, and I've never been scared at work before. I am scared that we will lose control," she said. "I cry every day when I walk in to work, and I cry every day when I walk to my car after work."[1]

COVID-19 shows that infectious diseases can be deadly. The staggering number of deaths from COVID-19 is significant; however, there have been even more lethal pandemics in the past. For instance, the Black Death—a plague outbreak during the 1300s—is believed to have destroyed half of the population of Europe. More recently, the 1918 influenza outbreak—also called the Spanish flu—killed more than 50 million people worldwide in just two years. Overall, infectious diseases such as plague, influenza, tuberculosis, smallpox, and human immunodeficiency virus (HIV) have wiped out tens of millions of people around the globe. In addition, they have left millions more suffering from chronic health problems or permanent disabilities.

Disruptive Threats That Rarely Disappear

However, infectious diseases have the power to do far more than kill. They also have a significant impact on the way society itself functions. Epidemiologist Michael T. Osterholm and author Mark Olshaker stress that infectious diseases are an especially deadly enemy because, unlike other types of illnesses, they strike society as a whole, disrupting and changing the way people live. They say, "Heart disease, cancer, even Alzheimer's, can have devastating individual effects, and research leading to cures is laudable. But these diseases don't really have the potential to alter the day-to-day functioning of society, halt travel, trade, and industry or foster political instability."[2] In contrast, infectious diseases have the power do all of these things, and a look at history shows that they often do.

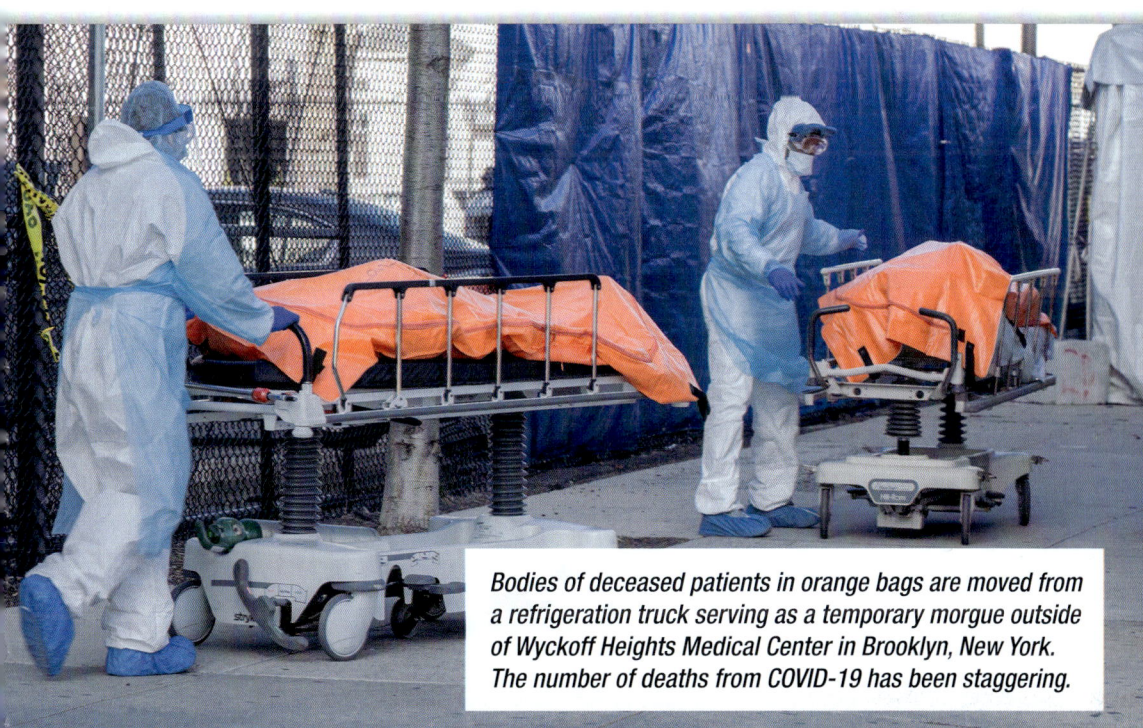

Bodies of deceased patients in orange bags are moved from a refrigeration truck serving as a temporary morgue outside of Wyckoff Heights Medical Center in Brooklyn, New York. The number of deaths from COVID-19 has been staggering.

Finally, deadly infectious diseases are a threat that never goes away. Throughout history, a long—and constantly changing—list of infectious diseases has continued to threaten populations all over the world. In fact, for most of history, infectious diseases were the most common way for people to die. For example, a hundred years ago influenza, tuberculosis, and diarrheal diseases were some of the most common causes of death. In recent years, medical advances have changed that in some places, and chronic diseases such as cancer, heart disease, and diabetes have overtaken infectious diseases as the leading causes of death worldwide. However, infectious diseases continue to be a major threat, and in low-income countries, people are still more likely to die of an infectious disease than anything else.

Overall, most experts agree that infectious diseases will continue to be a major health threat in the future. This is because existing diseases are extremely difficult to get rid of and because new diseases continually emerge. Despite extensive research and significant scientific advances in the fight against infectious diseases, society has only been able to eradicate two of them: smallpox and rinderpest. In contrast, the World Health Organization (WHO) estimates that at least thirty new infectious diseases have emerged just since the 1970s. When COVID-19 struck in 2019, many experts were not surprised because they had already predicted that it was just a matter of time until another deadly infectious disease caused a major pandemic. These same experts also warn that COVID-19 will not be the last deadly infectious disease to threaten society. According to medical historian Mark Honigsbaum, "Reviewing the last hundred years of epidemic outbreaks, the only thing that is certain is that there will be new plagues and new pandemics. It is not a question of if, we are told, but when. Pestilences may be unpredictable, but we should expect them to recur."[3]

pandemic

An infectious disease outbreak that occurs over multiple countries or continents and affects a large proportion of the population

CHAPTER ONE

About Infectious Diseases

In 2007 Rachel Futterman was a sophomore in college. A dancer and volleyball player, she planned to attend law school after she graduated. One day she woke up with a headache and told her friends that she felt like she might be coming down with the flu. However, when a roommate later came by to check on her, she found that Rachel had suddenly become so sick that she could not get out of bed. When she tried, she had a seizure and was rushed to the hospital, where doctors had to sedate her because she could not breathe properly. The National Meningitis Association (NMA) tells her story on its website, concluding, "Sadly, Rachel never woke up."[4] She died of meningococcal disease, also called meningitis, an infectious disease that causes swelling of the membranes around the brain and spinal cord. Meningitis is so deadly that it can kill within a day of symptoms first appearing. According to the NMA, out of every hundred people who get meningitis, ten to fifteen die, and many of those who survive suffer from long-term disabilities.

What Causes Infectious Disease?

Meningitis is just one of hundreds of different infectious diseases that exist around the world. As Rachel's story shows, infectious diseases can kill rapidly. They can also spread rapidly, killing hundreds of thousands of people in a short period

> **microorganism**
>
> A tiny living thing that can only be seen with a microscope

of time. Yet although the effects of infectious diseases can be big, all these diseases begin with something very small—a microorganism. Microorganisms are tiny living things that can only be seen with a microscope. They exist almost everywhere—in the air, the water, the ground, and even the human body—and they play a vital role in keeping the environment and the human body healthy. For instance, microorganisms in soil break down waste and keep the soil fertile, and microorganisms in the human intestine help digest food and protect the body from disease. Without microorganisms, life on Earth would not exist.

Most of the millions of microorganisms in the world do not cause any harm to people. However, some types of microorganisms cause disease. These are called pathogens. Infectious diseases are caused by pathogens that get into the body and make it sick. Some pathogens originate in the environment, in places such as the air, water, or ground. Anthrax is an infectious disease caused by bacteria that exist in soil, and it can cause ulcers on the skin and can be fatal if inhaled. A significant number of infectious diseases, though, come from animals rather than the environment. An example is severe acute respiratory syndrome (SARS), which caused a global outbreak in 2003, infecting more than eight thousand people and killing more than seven hundred. The SARS pathogen came from horseshoe bats in China.

Types of Pathogens

There are different types of disease-causing pathogens, including bacteria, viruses, fungi, and parasites. Bacteria are living organisms made of a single cell. When bacteria get into the human body, they can multiply quickly by splitting into copies of themselves and then spread throughout the body and make a person sick. Examples of infectious diseases caused by bacteria are tuberculosis and cholera. Bacterial infections are often treated with antibiotics, which attack the harmful bacterial cells and kill them or stop them from replicating. The first modern antibiotic, penicillin, was discovered by Alexander Fleming in 1928.

Viruses are some of the most common causes of infectious disease. These pathogens are not cellular creatures like bacteria; instead, they simply consist of proteins and genetic material. In fact, there is debate over whether viruses are living. Alive or not, viruses do need a living host to reproduce; thus, after they get inside the body, they take control of its cells and turn them into virus-making factories. COVID-19 and HIV are infectious diseases that are caused by viruses. Some viral infections can be treated with antiviral drugs that stop the virus from replicating.

Infectious diseases can also be caused by fungi and parasites. Fungi are microorganisms that reproduce and spread by releasing spores. People catch fungal infections by breathing spores into their lungs or by getting the spores on their skin. Ringworm is a fungal disease that causes an itchy skin rash. Like ringworm, most fungal infections are not life-threatening. Parasitic infections, in contrast, can be fatal. Parasites live on—or inside—a host body

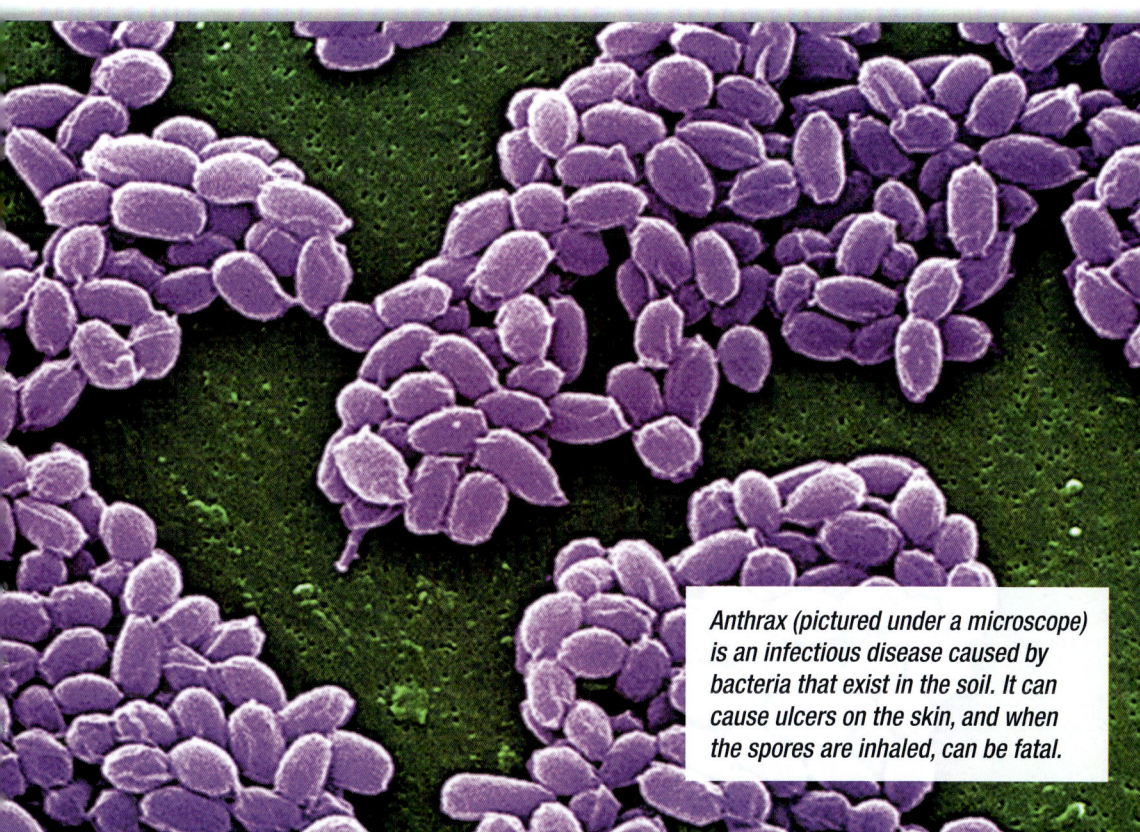

Anthrax (pictured under a microscope) is an infectious disease caused by bacteria that exist in the soil. It can cause ulcers on the skin, and when the spores are inhaled, can be fatal.

Infectious Diseases and "Waves"

Scientists discussing diseases sometimes mention "waves" of infection. For example, during the COVID-19 pandemic, there has been debate over whether the rate of infections will continually slow or whether there will be future waves of infections. The theory that some diseases recur in waves is based on the observation that when an infectious disease strikes a population, the number of infected often gradually increases, reaches a high point, and then recedes again, with a pattern that looks like an ocean wave. Experts propose theories about why infection might exhibit this behavior. Epidemiologist Abram L. Wagner explains that some infectious diseases follow seasonal patterns, spreading more quickly at certain times of the year: "Some pathogens may spread less well with greater humidity. Annual epidemics, like . . . influenza may occur because of climate or patterns of social mixing—often driven by the school year or people staying inside more during the winter." Waves might finally subside, according to Wagner, when enough of the population acquires immunity. He explains: "As more individuals become immune to a pathogen, its spread slows and eventually stops as the virus runs out of new people to infect." This is what is often referred to as *herd immunity*.

Abram L. Wagner, "What Makes a 'Wave' of Disease? An Epidemiologist Explains," The Conversation, July 6, 2020. https://theconversation.com.

and take their nutrients from that body. They can be as small as a single cell or large enough to be seen by the naked eye. Malaria is caused by a parasite that gets into the body through a mosquito bite and then multiplies inside the liver and the red blood cells.

How Infectious Diseases Spread

Infectious diseases spread in different ways, depending on the disease. You can catch some infectious diseases through direct contact with an infected person. These include touching, kissing, having sexual contact, or having contact with an infected person's bodily fluids, such as saliva or blood. Many infectious diseases spread when a sick person coughs or sneezes and infected droplets get into the air. Another person then becomes infected by breathing in those droplets or getting them on their hands and then rubbing them into their eyes, mouth, or nose. Tuberculosis spreads this way.

Some pathogens can stay alive for a certain amount of time on surfaces such as door handles or faucets, and people can catch them by touching those surfaces after an infected person has touched them. People can also catch infectious diseases through contact with food or water that is contaminated. For example, in countries that do not have adequate sewage disposal systems, drinking water can become contaminated with pathogens such as cholera, and people who drink that water can get sick. Infectious diseases are also spread through bites. Rabies, for example, can be transmitted by the bite of an animal that is infected. Other pathogens are carried by insects, known as vectors, and spread through bites. For example, mosquitoes carry several different infectious diseases, including dengue fever and malaria. Finally, in some cases, a mother can pass an infectious disease on to her unborn baby during pregnancy through the blood or other bodily fluids.

When the body is infected by a pathogen, the immune system fights back against it by making antibodies, which are proteins that fight off that pathogen. Sometimes, the immune system is not strong enough, and a person dies from an infection. However, in other cases, the immune system is able to defeat the pathogen, and some of those antibodies remain in the body even after the pathogen is destroyed. The next time the body encounters that same pathogen, it is better prepared to defeat it because it already has antibodies for that specific pathogen.

pathogen

A microorganism that causes disease

Researchers have developed vaccines based on this process. Vaccines train the body to fight a pathogen before a person becomes infected by it so that if he or she does later become infected, the body will be ready to successfully destroy the pathogen. Vaccines work in different ways, but one example is the measles, mumps, and rubella (MMR) vaccine. This vaccine contains small amounts of weakened or inactive virus. The virus in the vaccine is not strong enough to make a person sick; however, it stimulates the immune system to make antibodies to fight MMR pathogens.

Describing the Spread of Infectious Diseases

Infectious diseases spread easily through populations. However, not everyone who is exposed to an infectious pathogen will get sick from it. This is because every disease behaves differently. Some are extremely likely to spread from one person to another, while others are not. Researchers use a term called *reproductive number* or *R0* (pronounced "R naught") to describe exactly how contagious an infectious disease is. The R0 of a particular disease is the average number of people that one infected person will go on to infect. The higher the number, the more contagious the disease.

Scientists have utilized four key terms—*endemic*, *outbreak*, *epidemic*, and *pandemic*—to define how widespread a specific infectious disease has become. An infectious disease is termed *endemic* when it is almost always found in a certain area. For example, malaria is endemic to many African countries, meaning that it is an ongoing health problem there. An outbreak occurs when the number of cases of an infectious disease suddenly increases beyond what is normally expected in a specific area. This could mean

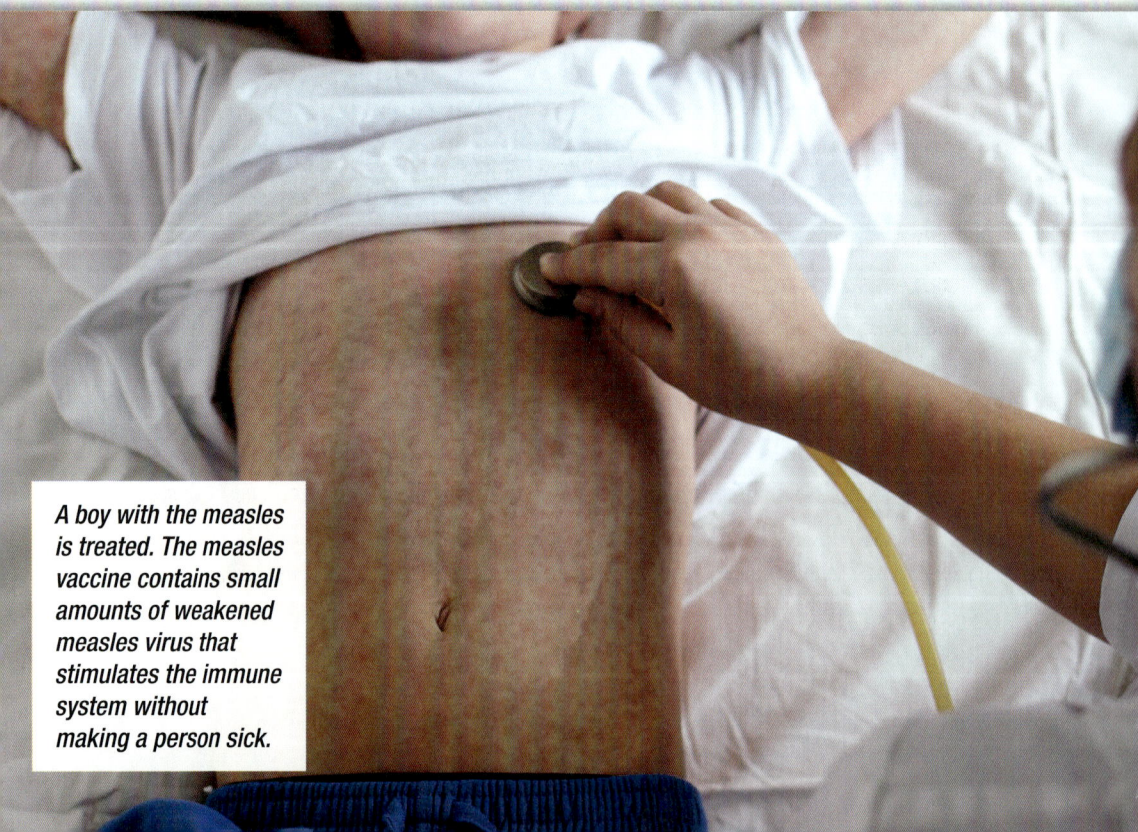

A boy with the measles is treated. The measles vaccine contains small amounts of weakened measles virus that stimulates the immune system without making a person sick.

an increase of cases in a region where a disease is endemic, or it could mean that an infectious disease shows up in an area where it has not been found before. In 2020 there was an outbreak of Ebola in the Democratic Republic of the Congo (DRC). According to WHO, it infected 119 people and killed 55. It did not spread beyond the DRC. An outbreak becomes an epidemic when it spreads quickly and unexpectedly to a large number of people in a relatively confined region. A Zika virus epidemic began in Brazil in 2015, with cases being reported in several other countries within the same year. A pandemic occurs when a disease spreads across multiple countries or continents. COVID-19, for example, is a pandemic because it spread to almost every part of the globe.

Higher-Risk Groups

Every infectious disease is unique, but in general, some groups of people have a greater risk of catching an infectious disease and are more likely to become very sick if they do. People with weakened immune systems or other existing health conditions are typically at higher risk because their bodies often have more trouble fighting off harmful pathogens. This includes those with illnesses that damage the immune system, such as HIV, or people undergoing a medical treatment that weakens the immune system, such as cancer treatment. Others at higher risk are the very young and the very old because they can have weaker immune systems. Finally, people with preexisting health conditions such as diabetes are often more vulnerable to infectious diseases because their bodies are already working hard to deal with these other health conditions.

However, infectious diseases do not always target these groups with greater ferocity. For example, although influenza is most often lethal to young children and the elderly, the 1918 influenza pandemic surprised doctors by killing large numbers of healthy, young adults. The COVID-19 pandemic has also surprised some experts by sickening a much smaller number of children than adults.

Socioeconomics and Risk

Although an infectious disease can strike anyone, regardless of social position or economic resources, researchers have found that people of lower socioeconomic status are often disproportionally harmed by epidemics and pandemics. Writing in the *Harvard Primary Care Blog*, physicians Rebekah L. Rollston and Sandro Galea explain that "socioeconomic status affects where we live, what we eat, what type of job we have, and whether we have access to health insurance and high-quality healthcare. All of this, in turn, determines our health." For instance, during the COVID-19 pandemic, people of lower socioeconomic status have had a higher risk of becoming sick because they often perform labor-intensive jobs that cannot be done remotely or they do not have the financial resources to stay home from work. Andrea Arcangeli is a taxi driver in Rome, and he earns the equivalent of about twenty dollars a day. He has two children to support and is unable to stay home to avoid coming in contact with the disease. "I have got a mortgage, bills and groceries to pay," he says. "I can't stay home." Unfortunately, driving strangers around in a taxi puts him at a higher risk of being exposed to COVID-19. Other low-income workers face the same predicament.

Rebekah L. Rollston and Sandro Galea, "The Coronavirus Does Discriminate: How Social Conditions Are Shaping the COVID-19 Pandemic," *Harvard Primary Care Blog*, May 5, 2020. http://info.primarycare.hms.harvard.edu.

Quoted in Max Fisher and Emma Bubola, "As Coronavirus Deepens Inequality, Inequality Worsens Its Spread," *New York Times*, March 15, 2020. www.nytimes.com.

Preventing Infectious Diseases

Because infectious diseases can be so disruptive and so deadly, throughout history people have been trying to figure out the best way to prevent their spread. Frank M. Snowden, professor emeritus of history and medicine at Yale University, explains that doctors during the Middle Ages believed that plague was spread through "fatal miasmatic smells" and wore clothing designed to repel these odors:

> People . . . tried to protect themselves with plague costumes, especially physicians, priests, and attendants whose duties brought them into contact with plague victims. . . . It was thought that dangerous atoms would not

adhere to leather trousers and gowns made of waxed fabric. A wide-brimmed hat could defend the head, and a mask with a protruding beak extending from the nose could carry aromatic herbs that would protect the wearer from the fatal miasmatic smells.[5]

Today, many people laugh at the idea of such a costume; at the time, however, many doctors took these costumes very seriously because they believed this was the best way to avoid getting sick.

Prevention strategies have changed over time, as researchers have gradually gained a better understanding about what causes infectious diseases, how they spread, and what stops them. For

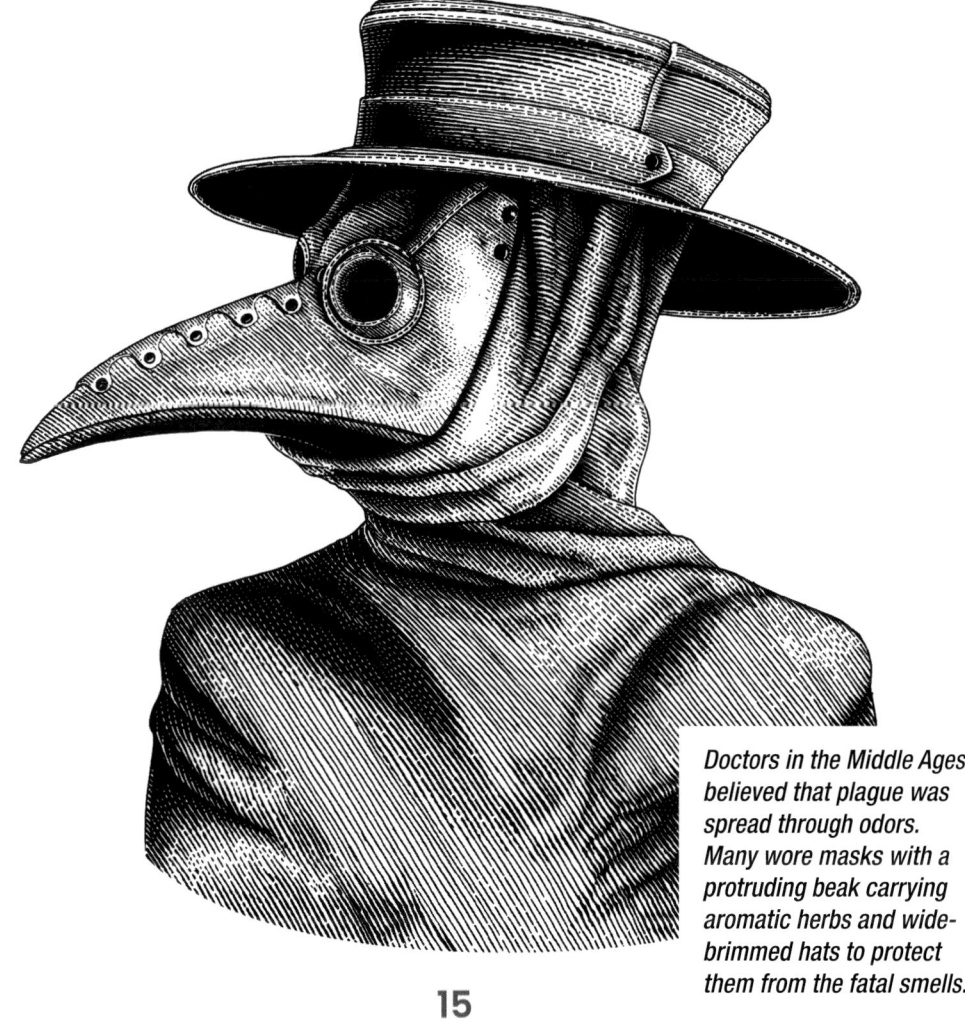

Doctors in the Middle Ages believed that plague was spread through odors. Many wore masks with a protruding beak carrying aromatic herbs and wide-brimmed hats to protect them from the fatal smells.

example, a major change in the fight against infectious diseases was the understanding that they are caused by microscopic pathogens and not things like "fatal miasmatic smells." The use of microscopes to study pathogens during the early nineteenth century ushered in the modern understanding of infectious diseases. Armed with an ever-expanding knowledge of the way pathogens spread and infect, medicine has been able to offer better ways to combat diseases. Today, society primarily deters the spread of infectious disease through improved sanitation and the distribution of public health information. When outbreaks occur, authorities impose quarantines while doctors ready antibiotics and vaccinations to halt the spread and reduce the severity of symptoms. Although pathogens remain a health risk for humanity, science has provided a means to counter, survive, and, in some cases, defeat infectious diseases.

CHAPTER TWO

Endemic Diseases

The Joint United Nations Programme on HIV/AIDS (UNAIDS) estimates that seventy-two thousand people died of acquired immunodeficiency syndrome (AIDS) in 2019 in South Africa. The year before, there were seventy-six thousand deaths, and the total for 2018 was even higher. About 20 percent of the population of South Africa is infected with HIV—the virus that causes AIDS—and tens of thousands die of it every year. HIV is an endemic disease in South Africa; this means it is always present and results in a similar number of deaths every year. However, when people think about deadly infectious diseases, they often picture those that strike unexpectedly. An example is the 2009 H1N1 flu—also called swine flu—that appeared in the United States and then quickly spread around the world, killing hundreds of thousands of people within a year. However, many infectious diseases are less dramatic but just as deadly; endemic diseases—such as HIV has become in many parts of Africa—do not just strike out of nowhere like H1N1 did, but they still kill steadily, year after year.

A particular infectious disease can be both endemic and nonendemic at the same time. One reason for this is that diseases can become endemic to some areas but not to others. For instance, cholera is endemic to more than fifty different countries, but the United States is not one of them. Cases of cholera could occur in the United States, but if cholera did suddenly start making people sick there, it would be considered an outbreak or an epidemic, not an endemic disease. Infectious diseases can also start out as epidemics or pandemics and then gradually become endemic. For example, COVID-19 struck unexpectedly in 2019, quickly infecting and killing large numbers of people; therefore, it is currently considered a pandemic. However, some experts warn that this virus may not go away and could instead become a lasting problem—or an endemic disease—in many parts of the world.

HIV/AIDS

HIV is one of the deadliest endemic infectious diseases in the world. It is a virus that attacks the immune system and eventually makes a person much more vulnerable to other infections. When the immune system becomes severely damaged in the later stage of HIV, a person is said to have AIDS. HIV spreads through contact with certain bodily fluids—blood, semen and preseminal fluid, rectal and vaginal fluids, and breast milk. It most commonly spreads when people have unprotected vaginal or anal sex or when they share needles or other drug-injecting equipment. It can also be passed along from a mother to her baby during nursing.

After a person is infected with HIV, he or she might initially have very mild symptoms, or even no symptoms at all, for years afterward. However, if the virus is not treated, HIV leads to AIDS. The symptoms of AIDS include weight loss, fevers, tiredness, diarrhea, swollen lymph nodes, sores on the mouth or genitals, and pneumonia. People with AIDS also get sick from opportunistic infections, which are infections they catch because their immune system is so weak. They can get so sick from these infections that they die. According to the HIV website of the US Department of Health and Human Services, without medication a person with AIDS usually only lives about a year.

HIV is now treatable. Yet when it was first identified in 1981, there was no treatment, and being diagnosed with this disease meant that a person would eventually die. Before effective antiretroviral treatments were developed in the mid-1990s, HIV killed millions of people around the world. There is still no cure for HIV, but antiretroviral therapy (ART) is an effective treatment. When people are treated with ART, it lowers the amount of HIV virus in their blood, preventing sickness and lowering the risk of transmitting the virus to other people. Providing access to ART in the United States has meant that fewer people die from the disease.

> **antiretroviral therapy**
>
> A type of treatment that stops a retrovirus, which is a virus that replicates by inserting a copy of its genetic information into a host cell

Even with treatment, life can be difficult because of the need to constantly take medication and also because of fear and discrimination from people who do not understand the disease. A man identified only as Karta experienced this. He says that his whole life changed after he was diagnosed with HIV. As he explains, "My colleagues started to distance themselves from me and the hospital I was about to start working at refused to hire me, after I disclosed my HIV status. In the end I had to leave my hometown to escape the shame and judgement."[6]

Unfortunately, unlike Karta, many people with HIV do not even have access to medication, which means that HIV still kills many people every year. WHO reports that millions of people with HIV do not even know they have it, and only about two-thirds have access to antiretroviral therapy. It estimates that 690,000 people died from HIV in 2019, and that, in total, the virus has killed 33 million people worldwide. In 2020, UNAIDS reported that among women of reproductive age worldwide, AIDS is the most common cause of death. The majority of HIV cases and HIV-related deaths occur in Africa, where the disease remains endemic in numerous countries.

Malaria

Malaria is another infectious disease that affects millions of people around the world. It is caused by single-celled parasites that are transmitted to people through the bite of an infected mosquito.

The parasite enters a person's blood through that bite and then travels to the liver, where it multiplies. The parasites eventually pass back into the bloodstream and into the red blood cells. There, they multiply again until they burst through the cell walls and spread to infect more red blood cells. In addition to mosquito bites, people can catch malaria through infected blood—for example, through a blood transfusion—or by sharing a needle with someone who is infected. Pregnant women can pass malaria on to their babies.

There are several different species of malaria parasites, and the symptoms of this disease can vary depending on the species that is present. In general, the initial symptoms of malaria often include a fever, chills, and headache. In severe cases, as malaria parasites multiply in the body, this disease can cause confusion, seizures, coma, organ failure, and death. For those people who survive, some types of malaria can cause relapses for years after infection. This disease is curable and preventable, but, as with HIV, not everyone has access to those drugs that can prevent or treat it.

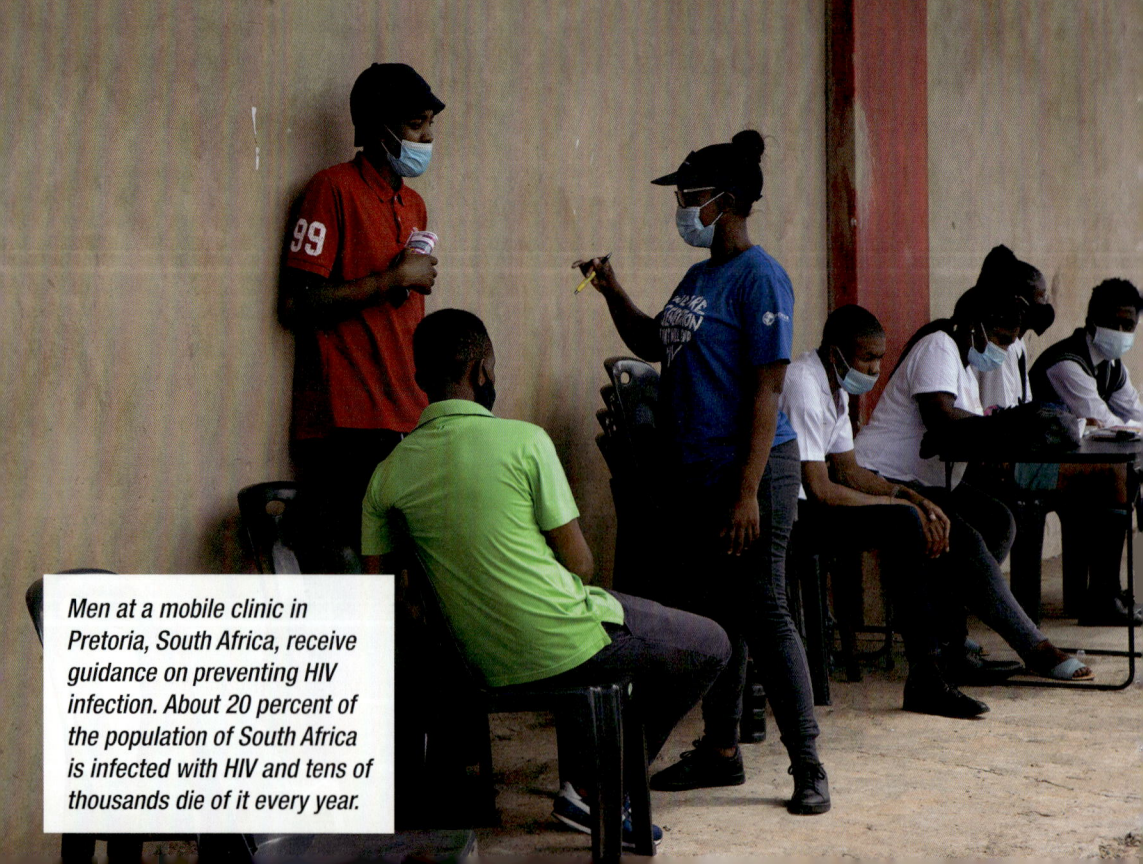

Men at a mobile clinic in Pretoria, South Africa, receive guidance on preventing HIV infection. About 20 percent of the population of South Africa is infected with HIV and tens of thousands die of it every year.

Rabies and Stories About Monsters

Rabies is a virus that spreads to people through bites or scratches from infected animals. According to WHO, the most common way people get it is from a dog bite. The virus is treatable if a person receives prompt medical attention after being bitten; however, waiting till symptoms appear usually means it is too late, and most people who wait that long do not survive. The later stages of rabies can include hallucinations, aggression, excessive salivation, muscle spasms, and delirium.

Jessica Wang, author of *Mad Dogs and Other New Yorkers*, believes that these horrifying symptoms may have inspired stories of werewolves and other monsters in the past: "The loss of bodily control and rationality triggered by rabies seemed like an assault on victims' basic humanity. From a real dreaded disease transmitted by animals emerged spine-tingling visions of supernatural forces that transferred malevolent animals' powers and turned people into monsters." According to the US Centers for Disease Control and Prevention, fifty-nine thousand people worldwide die from rabies each year. Rabies is a high-risk disease in China and parts of Southeast Asia. It is endemic to India, which has a large feral dog population.

Jessica Wang, "Rabies' Horrifying Symptoms Inspired Folktales of Humans Turned into Werewolves, Vampires and Other Monsters," The Conversation, October 29, 2019. https://theconversation.com.

Children are particularly vulnerable to malaria, and they account for many of the total malaria deaths that occur each year. WHO reports that more than half of all malaria deaths are children ages five or younger, confirming that a child dies of malaria every two minutes. A woman known as Augustine is a mother of four who lives in the town of Kintampo in Ghana. Her son, Philip, did not die from malaria, but he has been fighting it for four years. "It is very difficult for us all when the malaria comes back," she says. "He is very sick with fever, dizziness, diarrhoea, vomiting and headaches. He misses school often and I am worried about him falling behind his classmates."[7] In addition, she and her husband struggle to find the money to pay for treatment.

Because it is transmitted by mosquitoes, malaria occurs mainly in tropical and subtropical countries, where mosquitoes are abundant. According to WHO, malaria was endemic to eighty-seven countries in 2019. As with HIV, most of the world's cases of malaria

(94 percent) occur in Africa. Among African countries, Nigeria leads with 27 percent of the world's cases, and the DRC follows at 12 percent. Worldwide, malaria cases and deaths have both declined in recent years, but they are still significant. WHO reports that there were 229 million cases and 409,000 deaths in 2019.

Tuberculosis

Tuberculosis (TB) is another common infectious disease. Caused by bacteria, TB spreads when an infected person expels those bacteria into the air by coughing, sneezing, or spitting, and another person breathes it in. TB can affect any part of the body, but most often it affects the lungs. Although some people who become infected with TB show few symptoms, others get very sick. This disease can cause a long-lasting cough, chest pain, weakness, weight loss, chills, fevers, and night sweats, and it can make a person cough up blood and phlegm. Without treatment, it can be fatal. TB can be particularly harmful to people with HIV because their immune systems are weak. According to WHO, almost all HIV-positive people who get TB and are not treated will die.

Even with treatment, recovery from TB can be difficult. The illness is treated with antibacterial drugs, but getting better can take months or even years. Ingrid, a woman from South Africa who got sick with TB, describes how difficult her recovery was: "I was hospitalised for 75 days. During this time, I developed liver failure and nearly died. I woke up from the coma and the doctor said it was a miracle." She adds, "I remained weak when I left hospital and was struggling to cope with the injection and the pills that caused diarrhoea and vomiting. I found it hard to not have my freedom or the abilities I used to have, and felt very vulnerable and overwhelmed."[8]

TB kills many people all over the world. The Centers for Disease Control and Prevention (CDC) reports that before the discovery of the bacteria that cause TB, one out of every seven

> **antibacterial**
>
> Something that prevents bacteria from growing or spreading

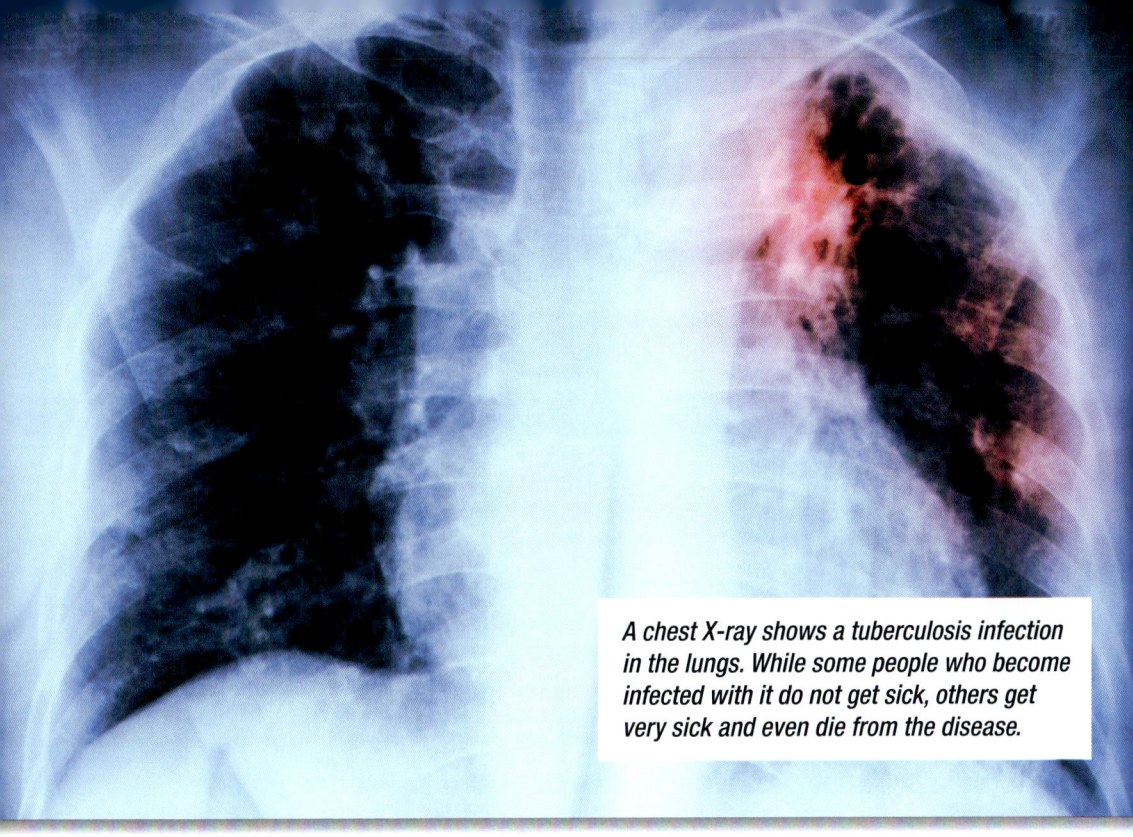

A chest X-ray shows a tuberculosis infection in the lungs. While some people who become infected with it do not get sick, others get very sick and even die from the disease.

people in the United States and Europe died of this disease. Even after the discovery of effective drugs, TB remains a deadly disease. According to WHO, 1.4 million people died from it in 2019, and TB remains one of the top ten causes of death worldwide. Thanks to treatment, it is no longer such a serious problem in the United States and Europe. However, the illness is still common in Southeast Asia and Africa and is endemic in thirty countries. WHO reports that in 2019, two-thirds of all new cases were in India, Indonesia, China, the Philippines, Pakistan, Nigeria, Bangladesh, and South Africa.

Cholera

Cholera is a diarrheal infection caused by bacteria. People become infected when they ingest contaminated food or water, and cholera often spreads in communities that do not have proper sanitation facilities or access to clean water. The symptoms of this disease appear hours to days after ingestion of the bacteria.

Infectious Diseases That Spread Through Sex

When people think about trying to protect themselves from infectious diseases, they often think about things like wearing a mask or sanitizing commonly touched surfaces. What they do not usually think about is sex. However, there are numerous infectious diseases that spread through sex—more than thirty according to WHO. WHO says that every day, more than 1 million people catch a sexually transmitted infection (STI). Some of the most common are chlamydia, gonorrhea, syphilis, herpes, hepatitis B, HIV, and human papillomavirus. Many STIs can be treated. However, WHO says that, overall, "STIs have a profound impact on sexual and reproductive health worldwide." For instance, they can cause pelvic inflammatory disease, infertility, and cancer. In women who are pregnant, they can result in stillbirths, and they can cause numerous health problems in babies that are born alive. One of the reasons STIs spread to so many people is that it is not always obvious when somebody has one. Yet even though they are not always obvious, a large percentage of people have been infected with STIs. According to the Centers for Disease Control and Prevention, one in five people in the United States has an STI.

World Health Organization, "Sexually Transmitted Infections (STIs)," June 14, 2019. www.who.int.

They can be mild, but some people who catch cholera get acute watery diarrhea, which can lead to severe dehydration and death. Cholera is treatable, and with treatment, most people will recover. Without treatment, though, a person can die within hours.

During the nineteenth century, when there was no known treatment for cholera, people were extremely afraid of it because of its gruesome and painful symptoms. Professor Snowden describes some of those symptoms. He says that extreme dehydration causes patients to resemble corpses: they are extremely cold and have sunken faces. In addition, he says, their blood becomes as thick as tar, and because it is too thick to properly circulate oxygen to the muscles, there is intense cramping. Snowden says, "The muscles contract in powerful cramps that sometimes tear both muscles and tendons and cause searing abdominal pain." Muscle cramps can also happen in the throat and can be severe enough to prevent swallowing and breathing, which causes the patient to suffocate. "Even after a patient dies," Snowden states, "cholera continues to horrify." He explains that "a ghoulish aspect of the disease is that, while the living patient resembles a corpse, the dead body of a victim seems alive. A haunting feature of the disease is that it produces vigorous postmortem muscular contractions that cause limbs to shake and twitch for a prolonged period."[9]

According to the CDC, cholera is endemic in fifty countries, most of which are in South Asia, Southeast Asia, and Africa. WHO reports that it infects 1.3 to 4 million people every year and kills up to 143,000. The organization stresses that although many people think of cholera as a disease of the past—and it is rare in high-income countries—it is still a serious problem in many lower-income areas that lack basic sanitation facilities.

A Heavy Public Health Burden

Around the world, endemic infectious diseases such as cholera kill hundreds of thousands of people every year, yet many people fail to understand just how deadly they are. Two researchers writing in the journal *Science* comment on how endemic diseases often become forgotten because they are less dramatic than epidemic ones. They state, "Epidemics . . . inspire decisive government investment and action, and individual and societal concern, sometimes bordering on panic. By contrast, endemic diseases . . . struggle to maintain the same attention."[10] Paradoxically, they say, although endemic diseases might provoke less concern, they are often a much larger burden to public health.

CHAPTER THREE

Epidemic and Pandemic Diseases

Ebola is one of the most feared infectious diseases. It strikes suddenly, is difficult to treat, and causes a painful death. Dr. Senga Omeonga is a surgeon at St. Joseph's Catholic Hospital in Monrovia, Liberia. He describes the horrific conditions that occurred when the hospital was overwhelmed during an Ebola outbreak in 2014. Omeonga also became sick in August of that year. As he recalls, "For one week I had my bed in the hallway. . . . At that time there was one toilet. But because a lot of people were using it—Ebola comes with the diarrhea—it overflowed and clogged. 'Poo poo' all over the floor." Instead of using toilets, he says, everybody was given a bucket. "So everybody has a small bucket for vomit, for everything," he explains. Omeonga goes on to describe the way that many patients did not even get the most basic care because the hospital staff were not equipped to deal with so many Ebola patients: "You're living like a nonhuman. . . . Sometimes you can have your bucket with you for all day [with] nobody to empty it. So you live in this area; the smell is all over. Sometimes you don't even have food because nobody [can] come in, [there are] not enough PPEs [personal protective equipment] to give to the staff. And you can scream all day of hunger."[11]

Whereas some infectious diseases—such as HIV—are endemic to certain areas and steadily infect a similar number of people year after year, others—such as Ebola—strike suddenly, and communities are often unprepared to deal with them. These types of infectious diseases are typically called epidemics. If epidemics spread across large geographical areas or even worldwide, they are called pandemics.

Plague

One of the most feared, notorious diseases in history is plague. This disease is caused by a bacterium that is usually found in rats and other small mammals. It is commonly transmitted to humans through the bite of fleas that live on these mammals. However, plague bacteria can also spread through droplets that an infected person breathes out or through contact with the bodily fluids of a person who is infected. Without treatment, a person infected with plague has a high chance of dying.

The symptoms of plague include chills, fever, fatigue, and muscle aches. Bubonic plague—the most common form of this illness—causes a person's lymph nodes to become hard and painful, sometimes swelling as big as a chicken egg. These swellings, or "buboes," can then turn into open, pus-filled sores. Plague can also get into the lungs, in which case it is called pneumonic plague, or into the bloodstream, called septicemic plague. Professor Snowden describes the agonizing symptoms of septicemia in his book *Epidemics and Society: From the Black Death to the Present*:

> The systemic infection initiates multiple organ failure. At this point patients have wild bloodshot eyes, black tongues, and pale, wasted faces with poor coordination of the facial muscles. They experience general prostration, teeth-shattering chills, respiratory distress, and a high fever. . . . In addition there is progressive neurological damage manifested by slurred speech, tremors in the limbs, a staggering gait, seizures, and psychic disturbances ending in delirium, coma, and death.[12]

Overall, numerous plague outbreaks have struck throughout history, and this disease has killed tens of millions of people. Researchers frequently focus on three major pandemics though. The first is the Justinian plague (named after Emperor Justinian of the Eastern Roman Empire), which occurred during the sixth century, spreading from central Africa to Egypt and the Mediterranean. It killed between 30 and 50 million people. The next major pandemic was the Black Death, which began in Sicily in 1347. The Black Death is the most well-known outbreak of plague in history. Heather E. Quinlan, the author of *Plagues, Pandemics and Viruses*, writes that it killed 70 to 200 million people. As she explains, "That's equal to between 30 to 60 percent of Europe's population. It killed so many that it took more than two centuries for the world's population to recover."[13] The third major plague pandemic occurred in 1894, beginning in China and spreading throughout the world. It also killed tens of millions of people. That was the last plague pandemic in history. In 1894 a scientist discovered the bacteria responsible for this deadly disease, and later, researchers learned how to treat it with antibiotics.

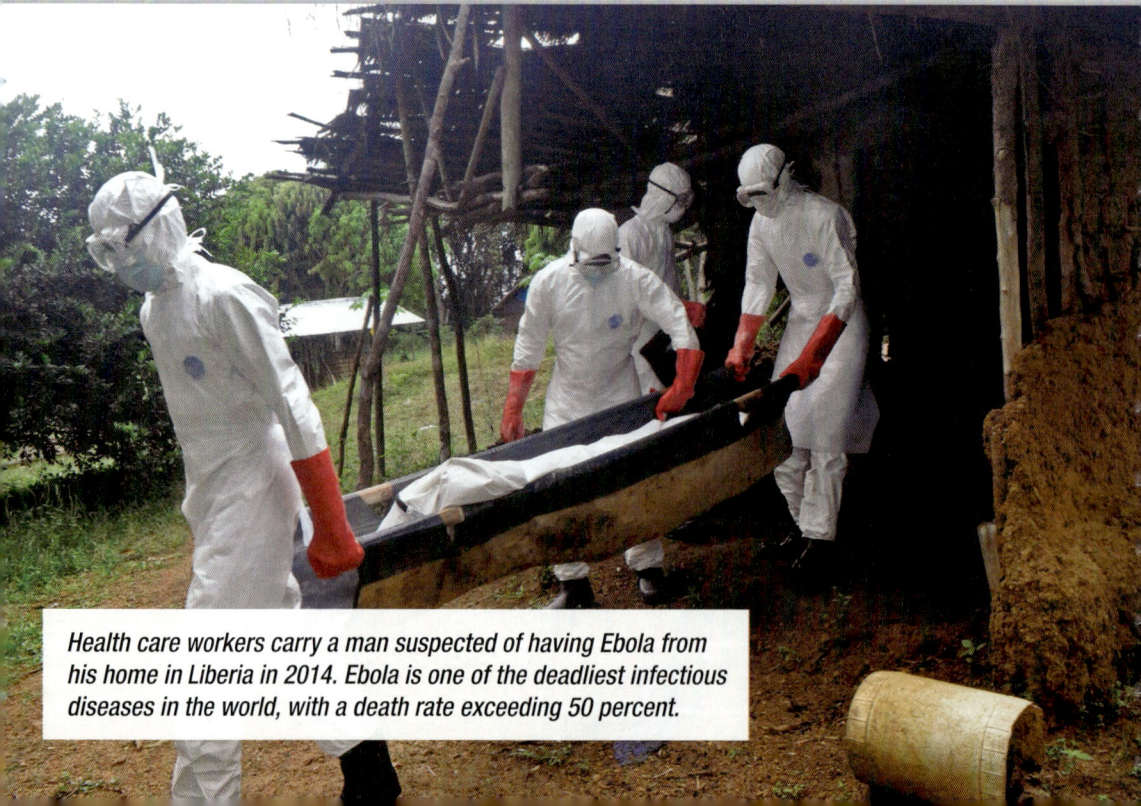

Health care workers carry a man suspected of having Ebola from his home in Liberia in 2014. Ebola is one of the deadliest infectious diseases in the world, with a death rate exceeding 50 percent.

Because treatment now exists, huge plague outbreaks are a thing of the past, but cases of plague still occur. WHO reports that plague exists on every continent but Oceania. In recent years, most cases have been in Africa, and the overall number is small. Today, plague deaths number in the hundreds, not the hundreds of thousands.

The 1918 Influenza

Influenza—or the flu—is caused by a virus, and flu outbreaks are a common occurrence in most parts of the world. There are multiple strains of flu virus, and they constantly change and evolve. The strain that makes people sick one year is different than the one that will arise the next year. Overall, most flu strains do kill people but not in large numbers. However, throughout history there have been some influenza strains that were particularly deadly. The 1918 influenza was such a strain. Sometimes referred to as the Spanish flu (because people falsely believed that it started in Spain), the 1918 flu caused a worldwide pandemic that killed tens of millions of people and dramatically changed life for many more. Researchers are not sure where this flu started, but cases were reported early in the United States, Europe, and Asia, and the illness spread around the world within months.

The flu virus can spread rapidly because it is very contagious. It spreads when an infected person talks, sneezes, or coughs and sends infected droplets into the air, which are then breathed in by another person. The flu can also spread when a person touches something that an infected person has touched and then touches his or her own mouth, eyes, or nose. This illness affects the respiratory system. The symptoms of the 1918 flu—and most other flu outbreaks—came on suddenly and typically included a fever, cough, body aches, a headache, fatigue, and sometimes vomiting and diarrhea. Many people went on to develop pneumonia or other respiratory complications, which are what caused most deaths.

Laura Spinney is the author of *Pale Rider: The Spanish Flu of 1918 and How It Changed the World*. She gives more detail

> **secondary infection**
>
> An infection that occurs after a person has already been diagnosed with another infection, often occurring as a result of the first infection

about the symptoms of this disease: "The vast majority of those who fell sick recovered, but among the unlucky minority who did not . . . the disease took a grisly course. They began to have trouble breathing, and their faces turned a mahogany colour. The mahogany darkened to blue—an effect doctors dubbed 'heliotrope cyanosis'—and by the time they died they were black all over." She goes on to describe some of the less well-known symptoms. "The flu affected the entire constitution," she says. "Teeth and hair fell out. People reported dizziness, insomnia, loss of hearing or smell and blurred vision. There were psychiatric after-effects, notably 'melancholia' or what we might now call post-viral depression."[14]

Today many secondary flu infections, such as pneumonia, can be successfully treated with antibiotics; in 1918, however, antibiotics had not yet been discovered. Instead, health authorities focused on prevention by trying to isolate the sick, using

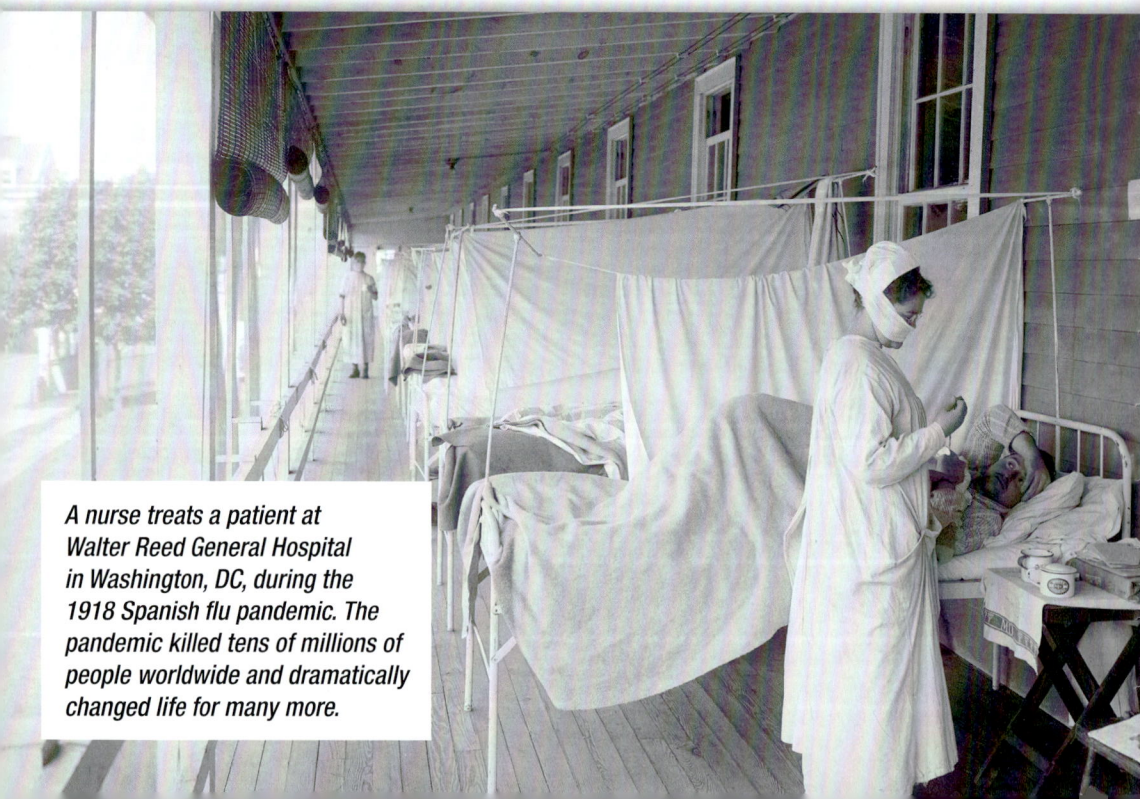

A nurse treats a patient at Walter Reed General Hospital in Washington, DC, during the 1918 Spanish flu pandemic. The pandemic killed tens of millions of people worldwide and dramatically changed life for many more.

The Disease That Paralyzed Thousands of Children

Every summer in the 1940s, parents across the United States lived in fear of their children catching an infectious disease called polio. Caused by a virus, polio can attack the central nervous system, causing paralysis and death. It most commonly appeared in young children and killed or paralyzed thousands of youngsters in the United States alone. David M. Oshinsky, the author of *Polio: An American Story*, talks about what it was like growing up at the height of the US polio epidemic when people still did not completely understand how the virus spread. "Each summer, polio would come like The Plague. Beaches and pools would close—because of the fear that the poliovirus was waterborne. Children had to stay away from crowds, so they often were banned from movie theaters, bowling alleys, and the like," he says. "Every stomach ache or stiffness caused a panic. Was it polio? I remember the awful photos of children on crutches, in wheelchairs and iron lungs. And coming back to school in September to see the empty desks where the children hadn't returned." A polio vaccine was discovered in 1953, and the last US case of polio was in 1979.

Quoted in Linton Weeks, "Defeating Polio, the Disease That Paralyzed America," *NPR History Dept.* (blog), NPR, April 10, 2015. www.npr.org.

---

disinfectants to sanitize, advising people to stay inside, and in some places limiting public gatherings and advising the wearing of masks. Many people still caught the disease and died. Unlike other influenza outbreaks, which typically kill a larger proportion of young children and the elderly, this one killed large numbers of young, healthy people. The CDC estimates that during the pandemic, 500 million people were infected—which was a third of the world's population—and 50 million died worldwide, with 675,000 deaths in the United States. WHO has called it "the single most devastating disease outbreak in human history."[15]

Ebola

Ebola is caused by a virus. Researchers are not sure where this virus comes from, but they believe it may originate in bats. It is transmitted to people through contact with the blood or other bodily fluids of infected animals. It then spreads from person to person through contact with bodily fluids such as blood, vomit, mucus, and breast milk. People can also get it through sexual contact. Five different strains of Ebola virus have been discovered: Zaire, Bundibugyo, Sudan, Reston, and Taï Forest. Each is named after the location where it was first identified. The Zaire strain has the highest fatality rate.

An Ebola infection often starts with a fever, aches, vomiting, and weakness. The virus interferes with how a person's blood clots, so it can lead to internal bleeding, which is why it is sometimes referred to as a hemorrhagic fever. Medical historian Mark Honigsbaum describes some of the symptoms of this notorious disease:

> Ebola hemorrhagic fever is one of the most virulent diseases known to man. It is also one of the most terrifying. One moment, victims are complaining of fever, headache and a sore throat; the next, they are doubled up with abdominal pain vomiting, and diarrhea. . . . The most alarming symptoms occur several days into the illness when cells infected by the Ebola virus attach themselves to the insides of blood vessels, causing bloody fluids to leak from the mouth, nose, anus, and vagina—even, on occasion from the eyes.[16]

Ebola is very difficult to treat and is often deadly. According to WHO, the fatality rate can be as high as 90 percent. Most Ebola outbreaks have occurred in Africa. The most recent one occurred between June and November 2020 in the DRC, where fifty-five people died.

Coronaviruses

Coronaviruses are a family of viruses that cause respiratory illnesses in humans. At present, seven different coronaviruses are known to sicken people. Four of the seven originated among animals. In fact, hundreds of coronaviruses exist in animal popula-

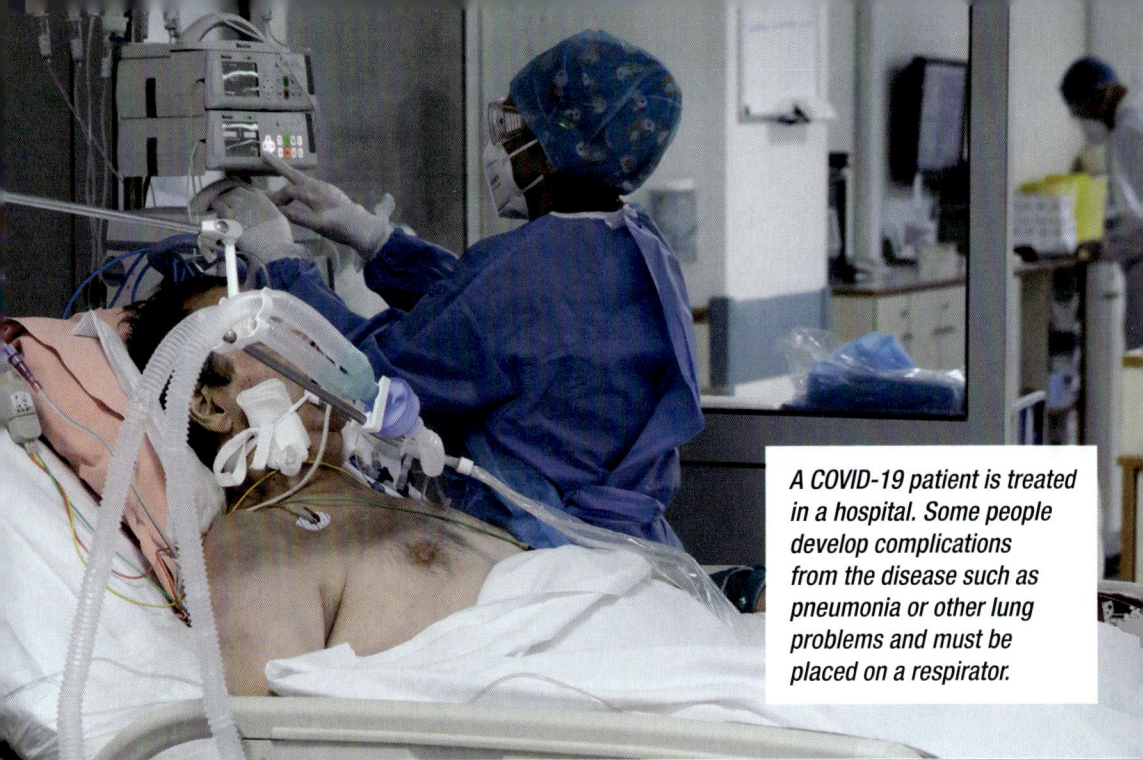

A COVID-19 patient is treated in a hospital. Some people develop complications from the disease such as pneumonia or other lung problems and must be placed on a respirator.

tions, but few cross over from animal into human populations and start to make people sick. COVID-19, however, is one of them, although researchers are still not sure exactly what type of animal it came from. *CO* stands for "corona," *VI* for "virus," *D* for "disease," and *19* for "2019," which is the year it was discovered. Since COVID-19 is a newly discovered virus, it is sometimes referred to as a *novel* coronavirus. One reason why new coronaviruses can be dangerous is because people have no immunity to them. This virus spreads when an infected person coughs, sneezes, or breathes droplets into the air and they are breathed in by another person. It can also spread when the virus is transmitted to an object such as a door handle and then another person touches that object and unthinkingly rubs his or her own mouth, nose, or eyes.

COVID-19 can cause a wide array of symptoms, including fever, cough, chills, aches, tiredness, shortness of breath, loss of taste and smell, headache, and

respiratory disease

A disease that affects the lungs and the airways that make up a person's respiratory system

Society Triumphs over Smallpox

Smallpox is one of only two diseases that society has been able to completely eradicate. However, before it was defeated, smallpox was one of the most feared of all infectious diseases. It caused sores to break out over the entire body, even in the eyes, on the soles of the feet, and in the mouth. These sores were hard and painful. Frank M. Snowden, author of *Epidemics and Society: From the Black Death to the Present*, writes that

> it was impossible for patients to drink, as even milk caused intense burning sensations in the throat. They experienced fearful weight loss and may have actually suffered from starvation. . . . The entire scalp sometimes became one large lesion entangled with hair. Pocks under the nails of the fingers and toes were a particular source of agony. The eyes became acutely sensitive; often they were themselves pocked.

Those who survived smallpox were often left with pits and scars over their bodies. Some went blind. Snowden estimates that during the eighteenth century, smallpox was responsible for a third of the deaths in children younger than ten years old and a tenth of all the deaths in Europe that century. It was eradicated in 1979.

Frank M. Snowden, *Epidemics and Society: From the Black Death to the Present*. New Haven, CT: Yale University Press, 2019, p. 94.

diarrhea. Some people develop complications such as pneumonia or other lung problems and must be hospitalized. These complications are the main cause of COVID-19 deaths. For people who are not hospitalized, COVID-19 symptoms often only last a few weeks, but there is also a significant percentage of people who continue to suffer from symptoms such as fatigue, difficulty concentrating, chest pain, and trouble sleeping for months after first catching the disease. In the United States, some people call them *long haulers*, and nobody understands exactly why their symptoms persist. *Atlantic* staff writer Ed Yong has spoken to many of these long haulers about how difficult COVID-19 has made their lives. He describes the case of Lauren Nichols: "She has lived through one month of hand tremors, three of fever, and four of night sweats," says Yong. "When we spoke on day 150, she was on her fifth month of gastrointestinal problems and severe morning nausea. She still has extreme fatigue, bulging veins, excessive bruising, an erratic heartbeat, short-term memory loss, gynecological problems, sensitivity to light and sounds, and brain fog."[17] Many other people echo Nichols's story of serious health complaints that linger long after they first become infected.

The first diagnosed case of COVID-19 in the United States was in mid-January 2020. According to the CDC, approximately a year later, there had been more than 25 million cases in the United States and almost 430,000 deaths. The Johns Hopkins Coronavirus Resource Center tracks coronavirus cases around the world. It reports more than 100 million cases and 2 million deaths in 192 countries.

COVID-19 is so deadly that drug companies and governments fast-tracked efforts to create a vaccine. The first COVID-19 vaccine was approved by the United Kingdom on December 3, 2020. The United States approved it on December 11. Several other countries followed, and additional vaccines were approved. Even as countries around the world began vaccinating their populations, authorities recognized that COVID-19 would remain a major problem for years and would likely not disappear.

CHAPTER FOUR

How Deadly Infectious Diseases Affect Society

Mary Beth Cochran lives in North Carolina. She takes care of her four grandchildren, who are between the ages of six and twelve. Like most children in the United States, they have been forced into remote learning because of the COVID-19 pandemic. Cochran says that not being able to attend school in person has left her grandchildren struggling. One of them has been so stressed that she has been pulling her eyelashes out as a nervous habit, and another is receiving warnings that he could be held back in school. "It's heart-wrenching,"[18] she says. Cochran is not alone in her frustration. Across the United States, young people, parents, teachers, and other experts are all worrying that there will be lingering educational, social, and emotional issues because of the lack of in-person classes. Betheny Gross is studying the impact of COVID-19 on education. She believes that it will not be easy to counter some of the harms that COVID-19 is causing young people. She warns, "I don't think we can just start school next fall and say, 'Everything's going to be OK.'"[19] As worries about remote schooling illustrate, deadly infectious diseases do more than just kill people. These diseases often completely alter the way society functions and can have substantial—and long-lasting—effects on its members.

Epidemics and Mental Health

When normal life is drastically altered by an infectious disease, the struggle to deal with that change can have a significant impact on a person's mental health. The COVID-19 pandemic is a good example of this. This pandemic has turned life upside down for many people, causing unemployment for some, forcing others to work or attend school from home, and discouraging in-person socializing with friends or even family. As a result, many people are struggling with a lack of human contact and are feeling stress over losing jobs, fearing getting sick, and worrying about the health of friends and family. All these concerns are taking a toll on mental health, and researchers note that more people are struggling with these issues. For example, in 2020 the Kaiser Family Foundation reported that more than one in three US adults had symptoms of anxiety or depressive disorder, compared to only about one in ten the year before. Mental health problems have increased in young people too. The CDC

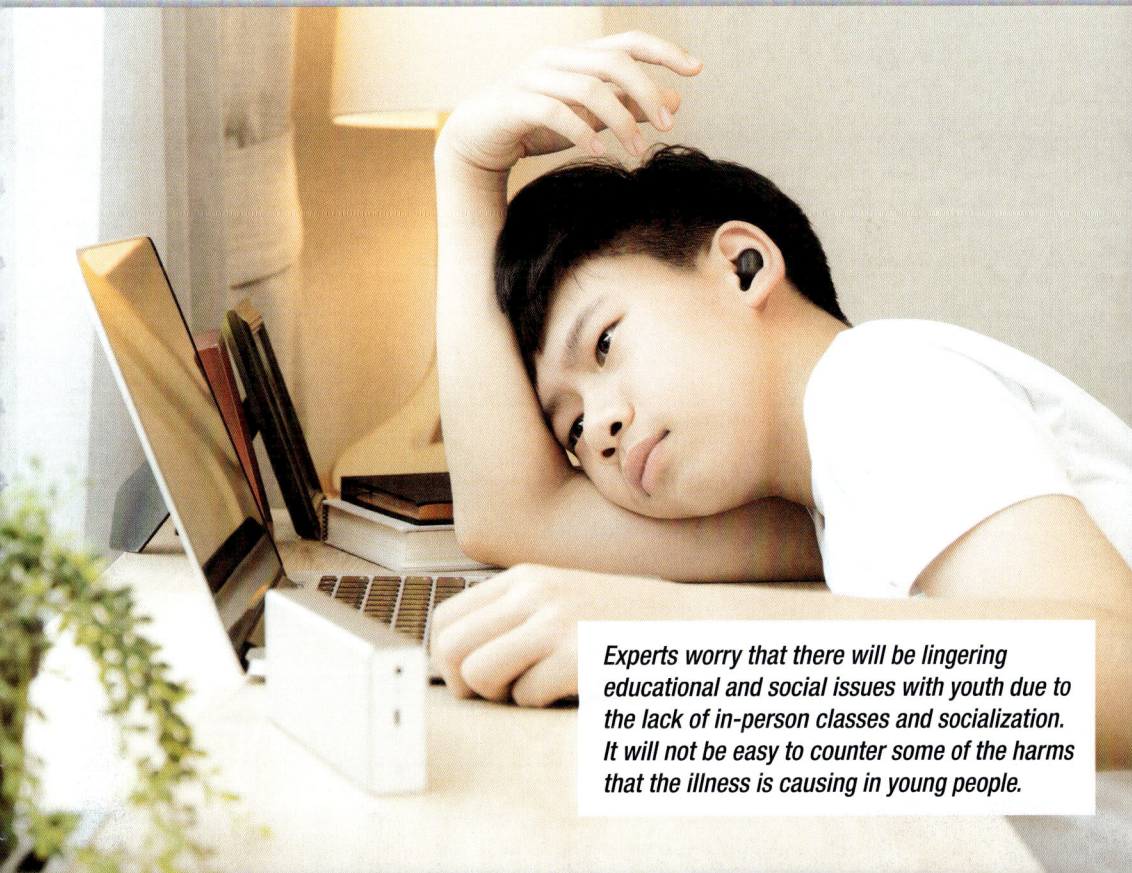

Experts worry that there will be lingering educational and social issues with youth due to the lack of in-person classes and socialization. It will not be easy to counter some of the harms that the illness is causing in young people.

finds that in 2020, children's mental health–related emergency room visits increased significantly compared to the previous year. Ayden Hufford, a teenager who lives in New York, explains how unhappy it makes him feel to be isolated from friends: "There's nothing to look forward to. On virtual days I sit on the computer for three hours, eat lunch, walk around a bit, sit for three hours, then end my day. It's all just a cycle."[20]

Yet even though many people say they are struggling with isolation and other changes that have come with the COVID-19 pandemic, others insist that not all the effects of COVID-19 have been negative. Many say that this pandemic has forced them to slow down, to spend more quality time with family, and to really think about what is important to them in life. For some, these things have made their lives better. As a young person in South Africa explains,

> The lockdown has made us realise the importance of actually appreciating the things and people that we take for granted. . . . It has come to show us that money and material things are not as important as human life and caring for each other in times of need, it has shown how much greatness can come from working together and what it can do for a nation and community just by giving a helping [hand] where it is needed and wanted.[21]

Some people worry that when the pandemic is over, their lives will actually become worse in some ways because they will be pushed back into their old routines that leave them too busy to take the time to help and appreciate others.

Racism and Xenophobia

Unfortunately, although infectious disease outbreaks can inspire people to help one another, they can also lead to racism and xenophobia. When an epidemic or pandemic strikes, life can change substantially; fear mounts as people become sick and die. History shows that fear often leads to the mistreatment of those who look or act differently. "This is a pattern we see again and again," says Amy Fairchild of Columbia University's Mailman School of Public Health. She explains that "it's 'the other,' the group not seen as part of the nation . . . that gets blamed for the disease."[22] For instance, when the Black Death struck Europe during the 1300s, Jewish people were frequently accused of poisoning wells or deliberately spreading the disease in other ways. An 1832 cholera outbreak in New York City was blamed on immigrants. Most recently, there have been reports of racist treatment of people of Asian descent during the COVID-19 pandemic because the disease was first reported in Wuhan, China. As Human Rights Watch notes, "In

xenophobia

A fear and hatred of foreigners or strangers

Fashion Trends Inspired by Infectious Diseases

Infectious diseases are usually associated with poor physical appearance. However, throughout history, some infectious diseases have caused major fashion trends. For instance, during the 1800s, TB—also referred to as consumption—inspired a fashion movement. Women with TB often looked extremely pale, thin, and delicate as they wasted away from the disease. When this look was romanticized by writers, many healthy women suddenly adopted the appearance of TB patients. According to Emily Mullin, a science writer for *Smithsonian*, "The height of this so-called consumptive chic came in the mid-1800s, when fashionable pointed corsets showed off low, waifish waists and voluminous skirts further emphasized women's narrow middles. Middle- and upper-class women also attempted to emulate the consumptive appearance by using makeup to lighten their skin, redden their lips and color their cheeks pink."

Another disease-inspired trend arose even earlier in history—in the seventeenth century—when it became popular for women to wear heavy white makeup on their faces. Images of Queen Elizabeth I display this white makeup, and her appearance is believed to have inspired the trend. Historians believe, though, that the queen used the makeup to cover the pockmark scars on her face that came from having almost died from smallpox when she was younger.

Emily Mullin, "How Tuberculosis Shaped Victorian Fashion," *Smithsonian Magazine*, May 10, 2016. www.smithsonianmag.com.

one typical incident, a Chinese-American reported 'I was on the phone with my mom speaking in Mandarin when a woman walked by and yelled "get this corona virus chink away from me," directed at me.'"[23]

The fear of others is not limited to racial groups. In many cases, recovered patients, as well as health care workers who have been in close contact with the sick, report that they have also been treated with suspicion or fear during epidemics and pandemics. Steven Taylor, the author of *The Psychology of Pandemics*, talks about the 2003 SARS outbreak and how some people were treated like they were contagious: "Survivors were even discriminated against and shunned, even though they had recovered. It's as if they were perpetually tainted. . . . There were reports of health care workers being told that their children were not welcome back into kindergarten because their parents worked with SARS patients in hospitals."[24]

Changing Social Norms

Infectious diseases can change behavior in many ways and then, when the threat of that disease is gone, people often return to living life as they did before. However, history shows that diseases can permanently change social norms and the way people behave. In some cases, these changes are relatively small. For instance, pandemics can permanently change the way people think about hygiene. During the 1918 influenza pandemic, people were told to sneeze into their elbows, cover their coughs, and not spit in the street because these measures would help stop the spread of germs. Following such rules is common practice today. Nisha Gopalan, a columnist who previously worked in Hong Kong, notes how hygiene habits acquired during the 2003 SARS outbreak are still in common practice. She says, "I still compulsively wash my hands, 17 years after the outbreak. I

> **social norms**
>
> The informal rules that govern behavior in groups and societies

Pandemics and Panic

As COVID-19 spread during 2020, it inspired panic around the world, and there were reports of people hoarding food and supplies. However, this is not the first time that a coronavirus has caused widespread panic. SARS, another disease caused by a coronavirus, became the first pandemic of the twenty-first century. It struck in 2003. Like COVID-19, SARS began in China and caused widespread panic as it quickly spread around the globe. Journalist Karl Taro Greenfeld was living in Hong Kong when SARS began. He talks about what he saw: "I recall going into a local Wellcome, one of Hong Kong's larger supermarket chains, to find the shelves stripped bare of toilet paper, ramen noodles, cooking oil, chili paste, canned soups, and, of course, rice." The panic over SARS led to mask wearing, stockpiling, travel restrictions, and quarantines, similar to the COVID-19 pandemic. Fortunately, SARS did not become as bad as many people feared. By isolating the sick, the world was able to stop the illness in less than a year. Overall, more than 8,000 people were infected, and 774 died. There have been no cases of SARS since then.

Karl Taro Greenfeld, "The Pattern That Epidemics Always Follow," *Atlantic*, March 5, 2020. www.theatlantic.com.

have friends that . . . use tissues to open the doors of public washrooms, or carry spare masks in their handbags in case they catch the sniffles."[25]

Other changes are much bigger than handwashing or wearing masks. An infectious disease can force changes in social norms that have life-altering consequences. Karestan Koenen, a professor of psychiatric epidemiology at the Harvard T.H. Chan School of Public Health, discusses the way that COVID-19 may be permanently changing the course of some people's lives. Koenen explains that the social distancing caused by COVID-19 is dramatically changing the way many people experience major life milestones such as graduation, getting a job, and dating. The result of these changes, she says, is that some people might live the rest of their lives differently than they would have without the imposition of those preventative measures. For instance, Koenen says, "for the older Gen-Zers: marriages, dating, jobs. . . . That's a formative period in their lives when people are figuring out: What's important to me? What do I want my life to look like compared to my parents' life?"[26] She says that experiencing these formative events differently is likely to forever change the way these Gen Zers think about the future.

The Economic Effects of Epidemics

In addition to changing the way people act and feel, an infectious disease usually has a significant impact on the economy, and that effect is often felt long after the disease subsides. Harvard University researchers writing for the International Monetary Fund explain the way that the economic effects of an infectious disease touch many parts of society. First, they state, "there are the costs to the health system, both public and private, of medical treatment of the infected and of outbreak control. A sizable outbreak can overwhelm the health system, limiting the capacity to deal with routine health issues and compounding the problem." They continue, explaining the way that the effects quickly spread beyond the health care system: "Epidemics force both the ill and their caretakers to miss work or be less effective at their jobs, driving down and disrupting productivity. Fear of infection can result in social distancing or closed schools, enterprises, commercial establishments, transportation, and public services—all of which disrupt economic and other socially valuable activity."[27] Finally, the researchers explain, the fear and disruption that often come with an infectious disease can last even after that disease is no longer a major problem; the result can be a reduction in tourism, trade, and foreign investment for years.

However, although the list of potential economic harms is long, past epidemics and pandemics have shown that when an infectious disease strikes, there can also be positive economic change. For instance, fatal epidemics or pandemics can kill so many people that they drastically alter the population, or they can change life so much that they cause people to question some of the things they have always done. The result can force a new way of doing things for the better. Stanford historian Walter Scheidel notes how pandemics lead to progressive change in

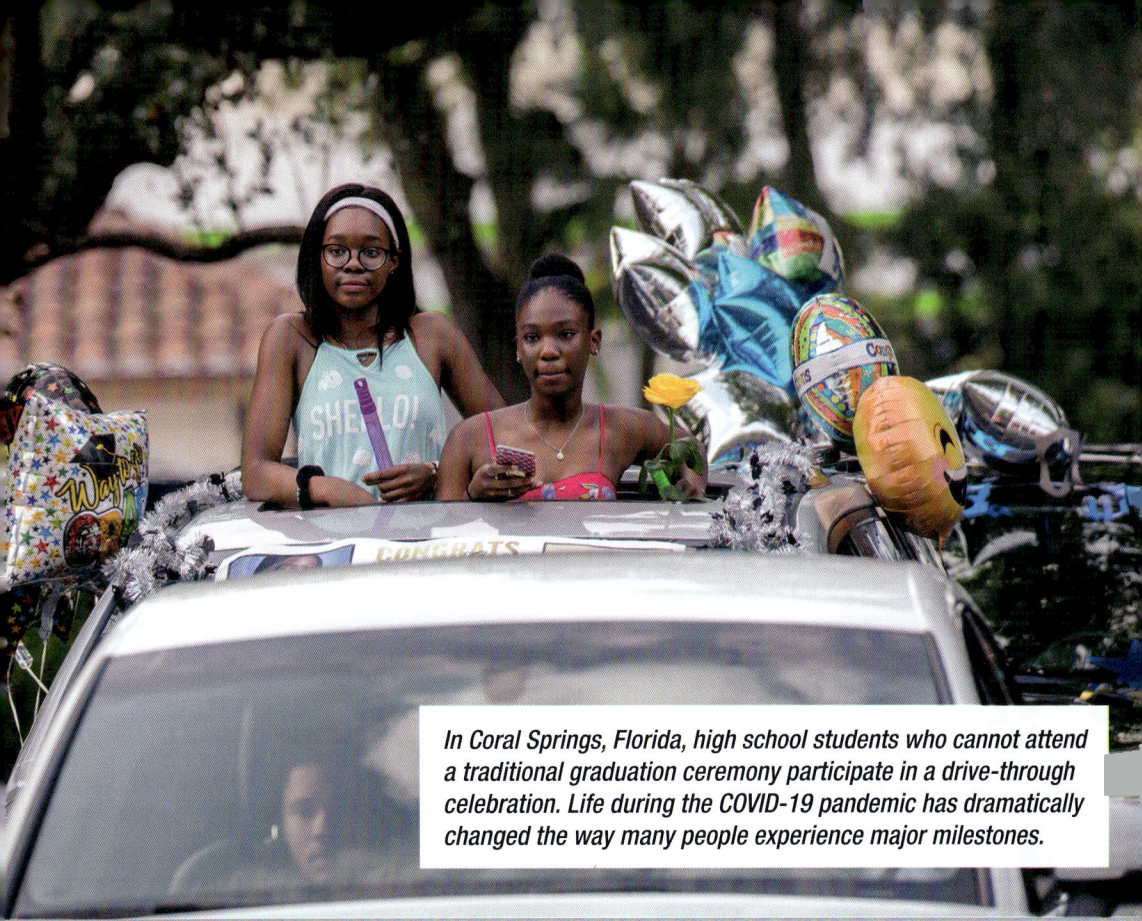

In Coral Springs, Florida, high school students who cannot attend a traditional graduation ceremony participate in a drive-through celebration. Life during the COVID-19 pandemic has dramatically changed the way many people experience major milestones.

society. He says that "throughout recorded history, the most dramatic and violent ruptures were also the most effective levelers of social and economic inequality: the collapse of states, the world wars, the great communist revolutions. The worst pandemics belong in the same category."[28] One of the best examples of this is the plague pandemic of the Middle Ages. Before the plague, a small number of landowners in Europe were in a position of great power, and most of Europe's people were poor laborers who worked under whatever conditions these landowners demanded. The peasants earned almost nothing for their work. The plague changed that because it killed so many people that labor suddenly became scarce. As a result, the laborers found that because the landowners needed them, they were able to demand more money and better working conditions, and their lives improved substantially.

Improvements to the Public Health System

Infectious diseases have also "benefited" society by prompting the discovery of new information about viruses and disease transmission and by inspiring communities to improve their public health systems. Hundreds of years ago, humanity did not have a good understanding of what caused infectious diseases and how to prevent them. Instead, when there was an outbreak of disease, people mostly just tried to keep away from the sick and waited until the outbreak was over. However, when outbreaks turned into epidemics and pandemics, and large numbers of people started dying, societies became more serious about finding ways to address the problem. Throughout history, the desire to prevent disease has pushed people to gain a greater understanding of infectious diseases and to develop better ways of preventing them. For instance, Professor Snowden explains that devastating plague outbreaks led to the appointment of public officials who had the power to make and enforce extraordinary measures to help reduce illness. "The new authorities were termed 'health magistrates.' . . . Originally, the health magistrates were temporary agencies, but by the end of the sixteenth century the cities in the vanguard of the war against the plague instituted permanent agencies, plague commissioners, and—as they were called ever more frequently—boards of health,"[29] Snowden says. One thing these new authorities did was to quarantine foreign ships to prevent them from infecting port communities. Boards of health and other official health agencies remain an important part of disease prevention today.

A more recent example of an infectious disease spurring improvements in public health is the 2003 SARS outbreak. Researcher Jennifer Bouey explains how the outbreak revealed weaknesses in China's health system, which made the country slow to recognize the outbreak and take action to prevent its spread. She says that recognition pushed the country to make substantial improvements: "SARS . . . prompted the country to rethink its approach to pandemic preparedness. The government soon invested 6.8 billion RMB (renminbi; $850 million) to construct a new three-tiered network of disease control and prevention systems."[30]

Sometimes society changes for the better and sometimes for the worse, but overall, infectious diseases do change the way people behave and how they respond to health crises. "Things are never the same after a pandemic as they were before," says Liam Fox, a former defense secretary for the United Kingdom, and he warns that "the current [COVID-19] outbreak will be no exception."[31] Society continues to speculate on exactly what changes might occur as a result of this most recent deadly infectious disease.

CHAPTER FIVE

Infectious Diseases in the Future

Throughout history, infectious diseases were among the most common ways that people died. That has changed. In 2020, WHO reported that seven of the ten leading causes of death worldwide are noncommunicable diseases. The mortality rates of infectious diseases, including malaria and HIV, have declined significantly. The top killer is now ischemic heart disease. Cancer and diabetes—also noncommunicable—are ranked in the top ten. Advances in sanitation and health care have helped society make a lot of progress against infectious diseases. Charles Kenny, a senior fellow at the Center for Global Development, says that "global efforts against infection over the past two centuries . . . have saved billions from premature death and billions more from stunted growth, pain, paralysis, blindness, or a lifetime of recurring fever." According to Kenny, "Two hundred years ago, almost half of all people born died before their fifth birthday, mostly from infection. Today, that figure is below *one in twenty-five*."[32]

However, this progress does not mean that infectious diseases are no longer a threat. In 2020, many nations were forced to a standstill and millions of people died as the COVID-19 pandemic ravaged the world. Hundreds of thousands of people still die every year from endemic infectious diseases such as TB and cholera. Overall, infectious diseases remain a significant threat, and most experts believe that threat is unlikely to disappear, despite continuing improvements in sanitation and medicine. However, although infectious diseases are likely to remain active, they are not likely to stay the same. History shows that infectious diseases are ever changing, with new ones emerging and old ones evolving. It is therefore likely that the nature of the threat of infectious diseases will continue to change in the future.

noncommunicable

A disease that is not transmitted through direct human contact

The Number of Threats Is Likely to Increase

Although infectious diseases might be losing their hold in WHO's top ten list, numerous researchers report that, overall, the number of infectious diseases and outbreaks are both increasing and will likely continue to do so in the future. As the National Academy of Medicine explains, "Much has been done . . . to mitigate the threat of infectious diseases to individuals and humanity as a whole. . . . However, despite these advances, we have in the last few decades seen several large-scale outbreaks of infectious diseases, not only old foes—such as cholera and yellow fever—but new threats such as Ebola, SARS, hantavirus, HIV, and novel strains of influenza." It warns, "We should anticipate a growing frequency of infectious disease threats to global security."[33]

The World Economic Forum also finds that epidemics have increased in number and diversity during the last thirty years, and it predicts that this trend will only intensify. Further, it maintains that in addition to global outbreaks, society should not underestimate the threat of smaller, more-localized outbreaks, which are also increasing in number:

> The risk of infectious disease can no longer be thought of exclusively in terms of rare but devastating events like global influenza pandemics. Potentially catastrophic outbreaks may only occur every few decades, but

highly disruptive regional and local outbreaks, such as the 2014 Ebola virus crisis in West Africa, are becoming more common and pose a major threat to lives and livelihoods.[34]

Antibiotic Resistance

One thing that helps infectious diseases remain a threat is the fact that they evolve. Experts believe that one of the most dangerous trends in the evolution of disease is that an increasing number of pathogens are becoming resistant to the antibiotics used to treat them. Antibiotics are important weapons in the fight against infectious disease. They are used to treat bacterial infections. In addition, even for illnesses caused by viruses, antibiotics are often used because people can develop bacterial complications to viral illnesses. For example, COVID-19 is caused by a virus, but its sufferers can develop bacterial lung infections. The 1918 influenza pandemic illustrates the value of antibiotics. That pandemic was deadly, killing millions of people. However, back then, antibiotics did not exist, and experts believe that a large percentage of those deaths were due to infections that could now be successfully treated with antibiotics. They argue that if the 1918 flu were to strike today, the number of deaths would be much lower due to antibiotic treatments.

Unfortunately, over time, some bacteria have evolved so that certain antibiotics no longer work on them. Overuse of antibiotics is believed to be one of the main reasons for this problem. WHO warns that "antibiotic resistance is rising to dangerously high levels in all parts of the world. New resistance mechanisms are emerging and spreading globally, threatening our ability to treat common infectious diseases." Furthermore, it states that "a growing list of infections—such as pneumonia, tuberculosis, blood poisoning, gonorrhoea, and foodborne diseases—are becoming harder, and sometimes impossible, to treat as antibiotics become less effective."[35] The CDC stresses, "Fighting this threat is a public health priority."[36]

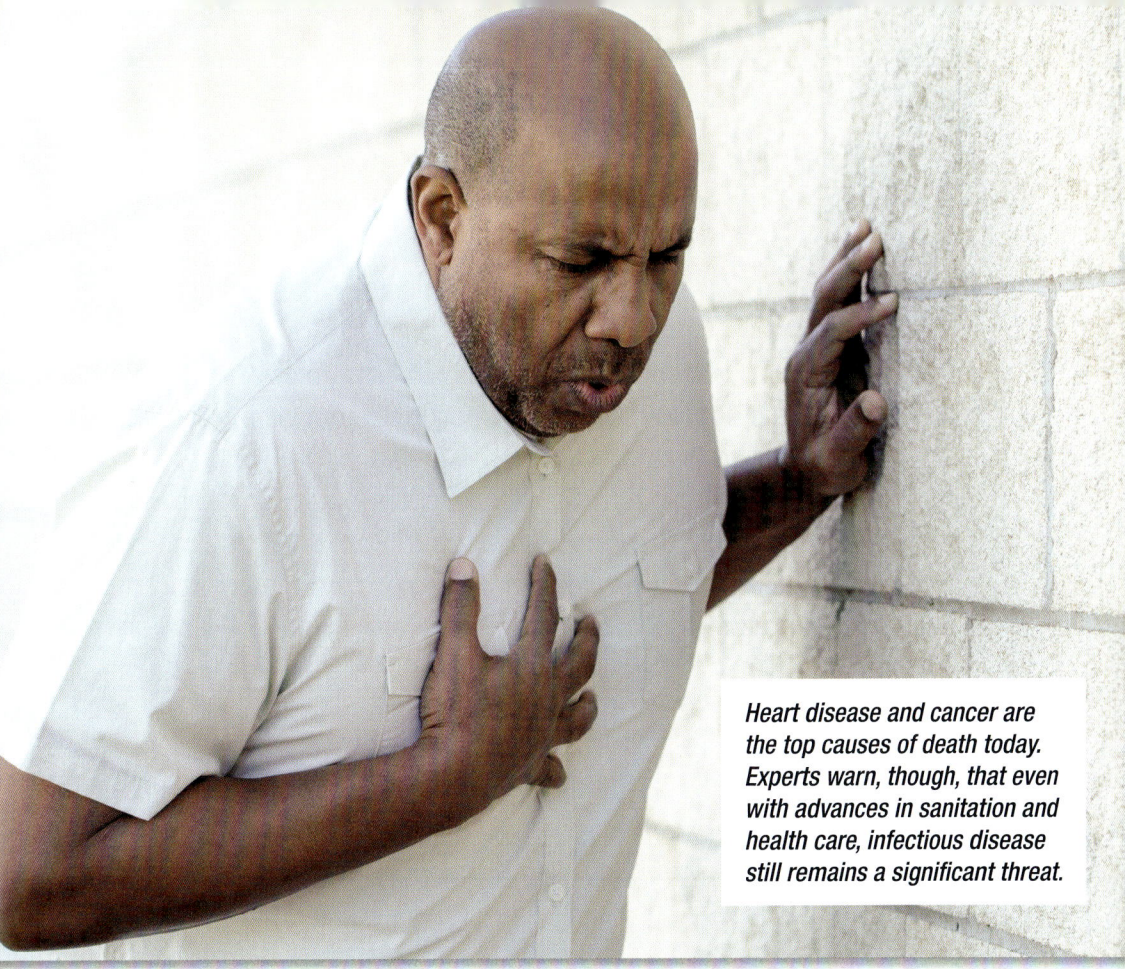

Heart disease and cancer are the top causes of death today. Experts warn, though, that even with advances in sanitation and health care, infectious disease still remains a significant threat.

Jay Propes suffered from an infection caused by a type of bacterium called methicillin-resistant *Staphylococcus aureus* (MRSA), which is resistant to the antibiotic methicillin. This resistance, he says, caused the MRSA infection to keep spreading. "With a history of lower back pain, I really thought nothing of it until I could no longer walk and even breathing brought excruciating pain," Propes says, "I was in a local hospital for 18 days. I had three surgeries in an attempt to excise the infection, but it just kept raging back."[37] Propes did eventually recover, but many people are not so lucky. The CDC reports that of those 2.8 million antibiotic-resistant infections that occur every year in the United States, more than 35,000 people die. Still, antibiotics remain an often-used defense because, without them, an infectious disease can be much more deadly.

Globalization and Population Growth

Another thing that is changing the nature of infectious disease is the way that society continues to become more connected than ever before. As global trade and travel increase year after year, it becomes easier for infectious diseases to quickly spread to large numbers of people. History shows that one of the main ways infectious diseases spread is when people move from one place to another. For example, plague spread along trade routes during the Middle Ages. Spanish explorers brought smallpox to Central America when they sailed there during the 1500s. Today, more people travel to more places in the world than ever before. For instance, according to data from the World Bank, 4.4 billion passengers traveled by air in 2019. In 1999—just twenty years earlier—there were only 1.6 billion air travelers. Johns Hopkins Medicine explains that all this travel allows infectious diseases to quickly spread far from where they begin: "With people's ability today to travel anywhere in the world within 36 hours or less, formerly little-known infections are picked up and rapidly spread to areas where they previously did not exist."[38]

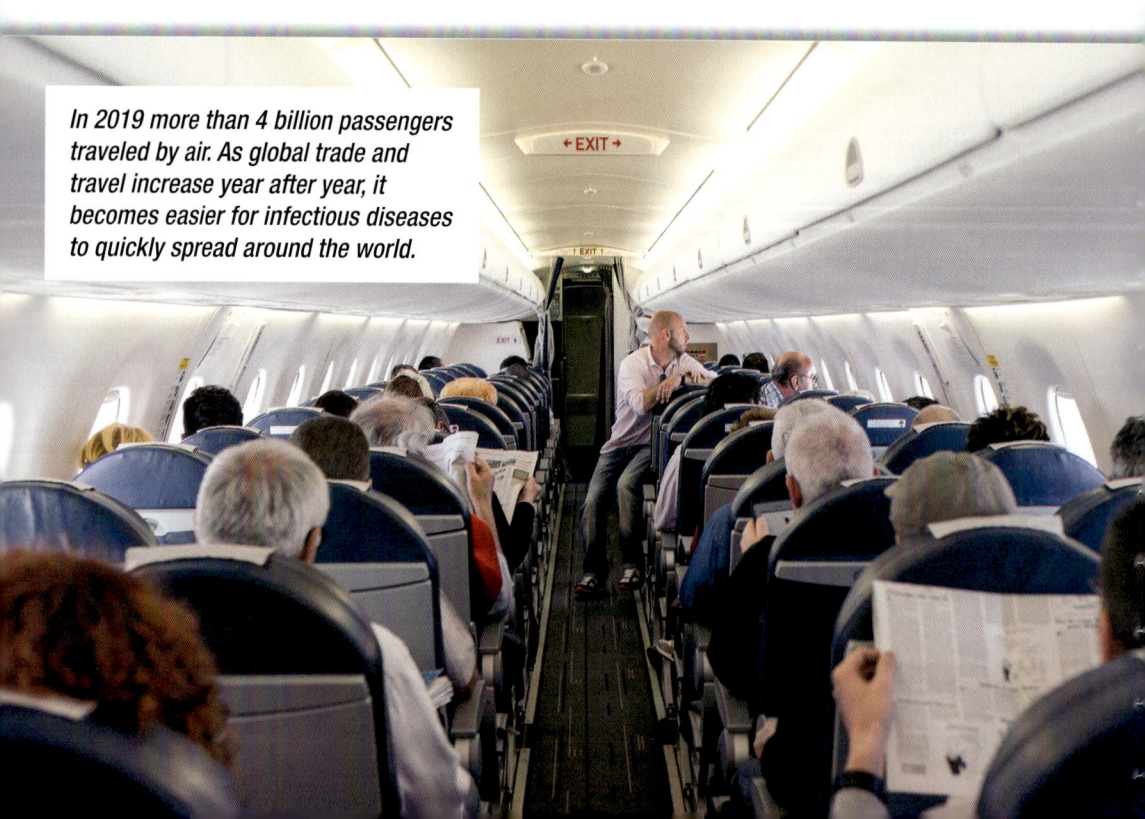

In 2019 more than 4 billion passengers traveled by air. As global trade and travel increase year after year, it becomes easier for infectious diseases to quickly spread around the world.

New Vaccine Technology

Over time, society has continued to get better at understanding and responding to infectious diseases. That includes improving the way it makes vaccines. In 2020 the United States and other countries approved the use of a new type of vaccine known as a messenger ribonucleic acid (mRNA) vaccine. The CDC explains how an mRNA vaccine is different from other vaccines:

> To trigger an immune response, many vaccines put a weakened or inactivated germ into our bodies. Not mRNA vaccines. Instead, they teach our cells how to make a protein—or even just a piece of a protein—that triggers an immune response inside our bodies. That immune response, which produces antibodies, is what protects us from getting infected if the real virus enters our bodies.

Whereas the traditional process of getting a weakened or inactivated germ can take a long time, the mRNA process is quicker to manufacture a vaccine. This first mRNA vaccine was approved to vaccinate people against COVID-19; however, many experts are optimistic that this vaccine technology may be used to create vaccines for many other infectious diseases in the future.

Centers for Disease Control and Prevention, "Understanding mRNA COVID-19 Vaccines," December 18, 2020. www.cdc.gov.

The growth of human populations is also changing infectious diseases by pushing human populations into closer contact with animals and their ecosystems. This increases the risk of infectious diseases because a significant percentage originate in animal populations. A disease that spreads from animals to humans is known as a zoonotic disease. For example, SARS is zoonotic. It is believed to have spread from animals to humans through wild game markets in China. As long as humans have an interest in capturing, taming, or eating wild animals, the potential for a disease to spread from the animal kingdom to humanity is increased.

Humans populations are also expanding into habitats where wild animals once

zoonotic disease

A disease that spreads from animals to humans

dominated. As animals and humans live closer together, and in greater competition for resources, the chance of contact between them increases, and so does the chance of a disease crossing from animal to human populations. The United Nations Environment Programme (UNEP) and the International Livestock Research Institute warn that "the frequency of pathogenic microorganisms jumping from other animals to people is increasing due to unsustainable human activities. Pandemics such as the COVID-19 outbreak are a predictable and predicted outcome of how people source and grow food, trade and consume animals, and alter environments."[39] According to UNEP, approximately 60 percent of human infections originate in animals. This organization and many others warn that zoonotic diseases will only increase as humans continue to expand their reach into nature.

Climate Change

The rapid growth of the world's population has also impacted the climate, and most people believe that climate change will, in turn, impact infectious diseases. Kieran Walsh, of the global health care organization BMJ Learning, argues that this is not just a prediction for the future but that the nature of infectious diseases is already being rapidly altered due to climate change. Walsh warns, "If you have any old books on tropical infectious diseases, then now might be a good time for a clear-out. The reason is that much of what has been taken as received wisdom in the past is now out of date. And the cause of this is climate change." For example, he says, "some of my old textbooks had maps of where certain tropical diseases might strike—but these maps are now being rapidly redrawn."[40]

There are a few specific ways that climate change can affect the nature and spread of infectious diseases. The Infectious Diseases Society of America (IDSA) explains three of the most significant. First, it says, if climate change causes rising sea levels and an increase in extreme weather events, the resulting flood-

The Threat of an Infectious Disease Bioterror Attack

A bioterror attack is the intentional release of infectious pathogens to make people sick. Some people worry that the next big epidemic will result from an act of bioterror. Epidemiologist Michael T. Osterholm has led numerous investigations into disease outbreaks. He and writer Mark Olshaker—authors of *Deadliest Enemy: Our War Against Killer Germs*—warn that there are many infectious pathogens in storage worldwide and that these pathogens are vulnerable to being transformed into weapons. In their opinion, the threat of a bioterror attack is very real.

They illustrate this argument using smallpox, one of history's most feared infectious diseases. Smallpox has been eradicated, but it still exists in research laboratories. Osterholm and Olshaker say smallpox would be easy to introduce into the general population, which has no immunity. The disease would spread quickly, causing widespread devastation while society struggled to understand what was happening, and how to stop it. They say, "There is no telling how many generations of spread we would go through before we finally had the crisis under control. Suffice it to say that it would overshadow 9/11 many times over and leave a permanent scar on the American and world psyche."

Michael T. Osterholm and Mark Olshaker, *Deadliest Enemy: Our War Against Killer Germs*. New York: Little, Brown, 2017, p. 139.

---

ing could damage water supply and sanitation systems, and this can lead to an increase in waterborne diseases. For example, the IDSA says, "in Haiti, recent hurricanes have severely damaged infrastructure and led to a large outbreak of cholera." Second, climate change could impact infectious diseases by changing natural habitats, which could alter the way some creatures behave. According to the IDSA, these changes could cause new infectious diseases to spread from animal to human populations or old ones to reemerge. For example, severe drought in Africa could force mosquitoes, which thrive near standing water, to seek water sources nearer to human communities. And third, climate change might cause warmer weather, which means that vectors such as mosquitoes and ticks are likely to spread to more areas, carrying with them infectious diseases. The IDSA explains that this is already happening:

> One example of this vector spread is the migration of the *Aedes aegypti* mosquito. Originally located only in the Southeast portion of the United States, this vector for the chikungunya, dengue, yellow fever, and Zika viruses has had its habitat extended into most of the mid-Atlantic and Midwest due to climate and weather changes, putting a significantly larger portion of the US at risk for potential outbreaks of these diseases.[41]

A Perpetual Challenge

Society has always been fighting infectious diseases, and although the nature of that fight might change, it is unlikely to end anytime soon. In an article for the *New England Journal of Medicine*'s two-hundredth anniversary, Anthony S. Fauci, the director of the National Institute of Allergy and Infectious Diseases, and David M. Morens, his senior adviser, write about the perpetual challenge of infectious diseases: "We will always confront new or reemerging infectious threats. . . . It is a battle that has been well fought for more than two centuries but that will almost certainly still be raging, in now-unimagined forms, two centuries from now." As Fauci and Morens stress, society should expect, and be ready, to always be challenged by deadly infectious diseases. They state, "The challenges are truly perpetual. Our response to these challenges must be perpetual as well."[42]

SOURCE NOTES

Introduction: An Ongoing Threat

1. Quoted in *Washington Post*, "What Seven ICU Nurses Want You to Know About the Battle Against Covid-19: Allison Wynes, 39," December 7, 2020. www.washingtonpost.com.
2. Michael T. Osterholm and Mark Olshaker, *Deadliest Enemy: Our War Against Killer Germs*. New York: Little, Brown, 2017, p. 4.
3. Mark Honigsbaum, *The Pandemic Century: One Hundred Years of Panic, Hysteria, and Hubris*. New York: W.W. Norton, 2019, pp. 367–68.

Chapter One: About Infectious Diseases

4. National Meningitis Association, "Tammy's Story." www.nmaus.org.
5. Frank M. Snowden, *Epidemics and Society: From the Black Death to the Present*. New Haven, CT: Yale University Press, 2019, pp. 61–62.

Chapter Two: Endemic Diseases

6. Quoted in Avert, "Karta: HIV Stigma Changed My Whole Life," April 15, 2020. www.avert.org.
7. Quoted in Malaria No More United Kingdom, "Augustine's Story." https://malarianomore.org.uk.
8. Quoted in World Health Organization, "Personal Stories from TB Survivors: My Journey Fighting TB: Ingrid, from South Africa," June 3, 2020. www.who.int.
9. Snowden, *Epidemics and Society*, pp. 237, 238.
10. Graham F. Medley and Anna Vassall, "When an Emerging Disease Becomes Endemic," *Science*, July 14, 2017. https://science.sciencemag.org.

Chapter Three: Epidemic and Pandemic Diseases

11. Quoted in Didrik Schanche and Sami Yenigun, "Ebola Survivor: 'You Feel Like . . . Maybe . . . a Ghost,'" *Goats and Soda* (blog), NPR, December 25, 2014. www.npr.org.

12. Snowden, *Epidemics and Society*, p. 47.
13. Heather E. Quinlan, *Plagues, Pandemics and Viruses: From the Plagues of Athens to COVID-19*. Canton, MI: Visible Ink, 2020, p. 42.
14. Laura Spinney, "The Flu That Transformed the 20th Century," BBC Future, October 17, 2018. www.bbc.com.
15. World Health Organization, "The Influenza Enigma," *Bulletin of the World Health Organization*, vol. 90, no. 4, April 2012. www.who.int.
16. Honigsbaum, *The Pandemic Century*, p. 280.
17. Ed Yong, "Long Haulers Are Redefining COVID-19," *Atlantic*, August 19, 2010. www.theatlantic.com.

Chapter Four: How Deadly Infectious Diseases Affect Society

18. Quoted in Erin Einhorn, "Covid Is Having a Devastating Impact on Children—and the Vaccine Won't Fix Everything," NBC News, December 15, 2020. www.nbcnews.com.
19. Quoted in Einhorn, "Covid Is Having a Devastating Impact on Children."
20. Quoted in Emma Goldberg, "Teen in Covid Isolation: 'I Felt Like I Was Suffocating,'" *New York Times,* November 12, 2020. www.nytimes.com.
21. Anita Mbenguzana, "Impact of COVID-19 in Our Lives," *Health* (blog), Voices of Youth, May 11, 2020. www.voicesofyouth.org.
22. Quoted in Brian Alexander, "Amid Swine Flu Outbreak, Racism Goes Viral," NBC News, May 1, 2009. www.nbcnews.com.
23. Human Rights Watch, "Covid-19 Fueling Anti-Asian Racism and Xenophobia Worldwide," May 12, 2020. www.hrw.org.
24. Quoted in Austa Somvichian-Clausen, "Why Outbreaks Like Coronavirus Drive Xenophobia and Racism—and What We Can Do About It," The Hill, March 5, 2020. https://thehill.com.
25. Nisha Gopalan, "Coronavirus: SARS Lessons Reduce Hong Kong Infection Rate," Bloomberg, March 6, 2020. www.bloomberg.com.
26. Quoted in Alvin Powell, "What Will the New Post-Pandemic Normal Look Like?" *Harvard* Gazette, November 24, 2020. https://news.harvard.edu.
27. David E. Bloom, Daniel Cadarette, and J.P. Sevilla, "Epidemics and Economics," *Finance & Development*, vol. 55, no. 2, June 2018. www.imf.org.
28. Quoted in Melissa De Witte, "Past Pandemics Redistributed Income Between the Rich and Poor, According to Stanford Historian," Stanford News, April 30, 2020. https://news.stanford.edu.

29. Snowden, *Epidemics and Society*, pp. 69–70.
30. Jennifer Bouey, "Strengthening China's Public Health Response System: From SARS to COVID-19," *American Journal of Public Health*, July 2020. https://ajph.aphapublications.org.
31. Quoted in The Week Staff, "How Pandemics Change Society," The Week, May 24, 2020. https://theweek.com.

Chapter Five: Infectious Diseases in the Future

32. Charles Kenny, *The Plague Cycle: The Unending War Between Humanity and Infectious Disease.* New York: Simon & Schuster, 2021, pp. 7–8.
33. National Academy of Medicine, Commission on a Global Health Risk Framework for the Future, *The Neglected Dimension of Global Security: A Framework to Counter Infectious Disease Crises*. Washington, DC: National Academy of Medicine, 2016. https://nam.edu.
34. World Economic Forum and Harvard Global Health Institute, "Outbreak Readiness and Business Impact Protecting Lives and Livelihoods Across the Global Economy." White Paper. Geneva: World Economic Forum, 2019. www3.weforum.org.
35. World Health Organization, "Antibiotic Resistance," July 31, 2020. www.who.int.
36. Centers for Disease Control and Prevention, "Antibiotic/Antimicrobial Resistance (AR/AMR)," July 20, 2020. www.cdc.gov/drugresistance/index.html.
37. Quoted in Texas Biomedical Research Institute, "Infectious Diseases Are on the Rise," July 17, 2018. www.txbiomed.org.
38. Johns Hopkins Medicine, "Emerging Infectious Diseases." www.hopkinsmedicine.org.
39. United Nations Environment Programme and International Livestock Research Institute, *Preventing the Next Pandemic: Zoonotic Diseases and How to Break the Train of Transmission*. Nairobi, Kenya: UNEP, 2020. www.unep.org.
40. Kieran Walsh, "Climate Change and Infectious Diseases: Now Might Be a Good Time for a Text Book Clear-Out," BMJ. www.bmj.com.
41. Infectious Diseases Society of America, "IDSA Policy on Preparing for the Infectious Diseases Complications Related to Climate Change," January 2019. www.idsociety.org.
42. Anthony S. Fauci and David M. Morens, "The Perpetual Challenge of Infectious Diseases," *New England Journal of Medicine*, February 2, 2012. www.nejm.org.

ORGANIZATIONS AND WEBSITES

Centers for Disease Control and Prevention (CDC)
www.cdc.gov

The CDC is the US agency responsible for protecting the health of the public. Its website has statistics, fact sheets, and reports about numerous aspects of infectious diseases, including causes, prevention, and prevalence.

Global Fund to Fight AIDS, Tuberculosis and Malaria
www.theglobalfund.org

The Global Fund is an international organization dedicated to ending AIDS, tuberculosis, and malaria. Its website contains news and information about these infectious diseases.

Infectious Diseases Society of America (IDSA)
www.idsociety.org

The IDSA is a community of over twelve thousand physicians, scientists, and public health experts who specialize in infectious diseases. It works to improve the health of people and communities by furthering research, education, and prevention efforts.

National Foundation for Infectious Diseases
www.nfid.org

The National Foundation for Infectious Diseases is a nonprofit organization that works to educate the public and medical professionals about infectious diseases to reduce the burden of these diseases. Its website has information about numerous infectious diseases and about immunization.

World Health Organization (WHO)
www.who.int

WHO is an agency of the United Nations that works to protect and improve the health of people worldwide. Created in 1948, the agency monitors and coordinates actions on many different health issues. Its website has numerous statistics, maps, and reports about infectious diseases.

FOR FURTHER RESEARCH

Books

Mark Honigsbaum, *The Pandemic Century: One Hundred Years of Panic, Hysteria, and Hubris*. New York: W.W. Norton, 2019.

Charles Kenny, *The Plague Cycle: The Unending War Between Humanity and Infectious Disease*. New York: Simon & Schuster, 2021.

Debora MacKenzie, *COVID-19: The Pandemic That Never Should Have Happened and How to Stop the Next One*. New York: Hachette, 2020.

Heather E. Quinlan, *Plagues, Pandemics and Viruses: From the Plagues of Athens to COVID-19*. Canton, MI: Visible Ink, 2020.

Frank M. Snowden, *Epidemics and Society: From the Black Death to the Present*. New Haven, CT: Yale University Press, 2019.

Internet Sources

Melissa De Witte, "Past Pandemics Redistributed Income Between the Rich and Poor, According to Stanford Historian," *Stanford News*, April 30, 2020. https://news.stanford.edu.

Human Rights Watch, "Covid-19 Fueling Anti-Asian Racism and Xenophobia Worldwide," May 12, 2020. www.hrw.org.

Alvin Powell, "What Will the New Post-Pandemic Normal Look Like?," *Harvard Gazette*, November 24, 2020. https://news.harvard.edu.

United Nations Environment Programme, "Preventing the Next Pandemic: Zoonotic Diseases and How to Break the Train of Transmission," 2020. www.unep.org.

World Health Organization, "Antibiotic Resistance," July 31, 2020. www.who.int.

Ed Yong, "Long Haulers Are Redefining COVID-19," *Atlantic*, August 19, 2010. www.theatlantic.com.

INDEX

Note: Boldface page numbers indicate illustrations.

acquired immunodeficiency syndrome (AIDS). *See* HIV/AIDS
animal habitats, 51–52, 53
anthrax, 8, **9**
antibacterial, defined, 22
antibiotics, 8–9, 48–49
antiretroviral therapy (ART), 18–19
Arcangeli, Andrea, 14
Asians, racism against and COVID-19, 39–40

bacteria, 8–9, 48–49
bioterrorism with infectious pathogens, 53
Black Death
　blamed on Jewish people, 39
　clothing as protection from, 14–15, **15**
　deaths from, 4, 28
Bouey, Jennifer, 44–45
Brazil (2015), 13
bubonic plague, 27

Centers for Disease Control and Prevention (CDC)
　annual rabies deaths, 21
　antibiotic resistance, 48
　cholera as endemic, 25
　infections and deaths from 1918 influenza (Spanish flu), 31
　number of COVID-19 cases in US, 35
　prevalence of STIs in US, 24
　seriousness of tuberculosis, 22–23
China
　COVID-19, 4
　1894 plague, 28
　rabies, 21
　SARS
　　origin, 8, 41
　　public health system, 44–45
　tuberculosis, 23

cholera
　appearance of corpses of cholera victims, 25
　cause, 8, 23
　climate change and, 53
　deaths from, 25
　as endemic and not endemic, 17–18
　New York City outbreak (1832), 39
　symptoms, 23–25
chronic diseases, deaths from, 6
climate changes, 52–54
clothing and Black Death, 14–15, **15**
Cochran, Mary Beth, 36
consumptive chic, 39
coronaviruses, 32–33
　See also COVID-19; SARS (severe acute respiratory syndrome)
COVID-19
　antibiotics and, 48
　cause, 9
　changes in social norms and, 41–42, **43**
　complications from, 34
　deaths from, 4, **5**, 34, 35
　first cases, 4
　impact
　　on education, 36, **37**
　　on mental health, 37–38
　　positive, 38
　long haulers, 34–35
　mRNA vaccines, 51
　naming of, 33
　number of cases in US, 35
　racism against Asians and, 39–40
　risk groups, 13, 14
　symptoms, 33
　vaccines for, 35, 51

Deadliest Enemy: Our War Against Killer Germs (Osterholm and Olshaker), 53
death(s)
　age at, 46
　AIDS in South Africa (2019), 17

60

Black Death, 4, 28
cholera, 25
chronic diseases, 6, 46
COVID-19, 4, **5**, 34, 35
Ebola, 32, 39
infectious diseases, 46
Justinian plague, 28
leading causes of, worldwide currently, 46
malaria, 21, 22
meningitis, 7
1918 influenza (Spanish flu), 4–5, 31
rabies, 21
SARS, 8, 41
smallpox, 34
tuberculosis, 22–23
Democratic Republic of the Congo (DRC), 13, 22, 32
dengue fever, 11

Ebola, **28**
    cause and transmission, 31–32
    conditions in Liberian hospital (2014), 26
    deaths from, 32, 39
    outbreak in Democratic Republic of the Congo (2020), 13, 32
    strains, 39
economics, 42–43
education, impact of COVID-19 on, 36, **37**
1894 plague, 28
Elizabeth I (queen of England), 39
endemic, defined, 12
endemic diseases
    cholera, 17–18, 25
    government action and, 25
    HIV in South Africa, 17
    malaria as, 21
    rabies as, 21
Epidemics and Society: From the Black Death to the Present (Snowden), 27, 34

Fairchild, Amy, 39
fashion, disease-inspired, 39
Fauci, Anthony S., 54
Fleming, Alexander, 9
Fox, Liam, 45
fungi, 9
Futterman, Rachel, 7

Gopalan, Nisha, 40–41
Greenfeld, Karl Taro, 41
Gross, Betheny, 36

Haiti, 53
Harvard Primary Care Blog, 14
health systems, 42, 44–45
heart disease, 46
herd immunity, 10
HIV/AIDS
    AIDS, 17, 18
    basic facts about, 18
    cause of, 9
    HIV
        cause, 9
        diagnosis of, 19
        immune system, 13, 22
        infections in South Africa, 17, **20**
        treatment of, 18–19
hoarding, 41
H1N1 flu (swine flu), 17
Hong Kong, 40–41
Honigsbaum, Mark, 6, 32
Hufford, Ayden, 38
human immunodeficiency virus (HIV). *See* HIV/AIDS
Human Rights Watch, 39–40
hygiene changes, 40–41

immune system
    HIV, 13, 22
    new coronaviruses and, 33
    pathogens and, 11
    risk of infection and, 13
India, rabies in, 21
infectious diseases
    as cause of death, 6, 46
    changes in, 47
    effect on society, 5
    evolution of, 48
    in future, 54
    risk of, 13–14
    spread of, 12, 50, **50**
    waves of, 10
Infectious Diseases Society of America (IDSA), 52–53, 54
International Livestock Research Institute, 52
ischemic heart disease, 46

Johns Hopkins Coronavirus Resource Center, 35

Johns Hopkins Medicine, 50
Joint United Nations Programme on HIV/
   AIDS (UNAIDS), 17, 19
Justinian plague, 28

Kaiser Family Foundation, 37
Kenny, Charles, 46
Koenen, Karestan, 41–42

long haulers, 34–35

Mad Dogs and Other New Yorkers
   (Wang), 21
malaria
   cause and spread of, 10, 11, 19–20
   deaths from, 21, 22
   as endemic disease, 12, 21
   prevalence of, 22
   symptoms of, 20
   treatment, 20
measles, **12**
measles, mumps, and rubella (MMR)
   vaccine, 11
meningitis (meningococcal disease), 7
mental health, impact of COVID-19 on,
   37–38
methicillin-resistant *Staphylococcus
   aureus* (MRSA), 49
microorganisms, basic facts about, 8
microscopes, 16
Morens, David M., 54
mosquitoes, 11, 19–20, 53–54
mRNA vaccines, 51
MRSA (methicillin-resistant
   Staphylococcus aureus), 49
Mullin, Emily, 39

National Academy of Medicine, 47
National Meningitis Association (NMA), 7
New England Journal of Medicine, 54
New York City, 39
Nichols, Lauren, 34–35
Nigeria, 22
1918 influenza (Spanish flu)
   antibiotics and, 48
   deaths, 4–5, 31
   hygiene changes as result, 40
   pandemic, 29–31, **30**
noncommunicable diseases, 46, 47

Olshaker, Mark, 5, 53
Omeonga, Senga, 26
Osterholm, Michael T., 5, 53

*Pale Rider: The Spanish Flu of 1918 and
   How It Changed the World* (Spinney),
   29
pandemic, defined, 6, 27
panic, 41
parasites, 9–10
pathogens
   antibiotic resistance, 48–49
   basic facts about, 8
   bioterrorism and, 53
   defined, 11
   immune system and, 11
   microscopes and study of, 16
   types of, 8–10
penicillin, 9
plague
   basic facts about, 27
   Black Death
      blamed on Jewish people, 39
      clothing as protection from, 14–15, **15**
      deaths from, 4, 28
      economic changes as result of, 43
      establishment of public health systems
         and, 44
      Middle Ages protection against, 14–15
   outbreaks, 28
   prevalence, 29
   spread of, 50
Plagues, Pandemics and Viruses
   (Quinlan), 28
prevention strategies, 14–15, **15**, 40–41
Propes, Jay, 49
Psychology of Pandemics, The (Taylor),
   40
public health systems, 42, 44–45

Quinlan, Heather E., 28

rabies, 21
racism, 38–40
reproductive number (R0), 12
respiratory disease, defined, 33
rinderpest, 6
ringworm, 9
Rollston, Rebekah L., 14

SARS (severe acute respiratory syndrome)
  changes in social norms in Hong Kong and, 40–41
  deaths from, 8, 41
  discrimination during, 40
  improvements in China's public health system, 44–45
  origin of, 8
  prevalence, 41
  as zoonotic disease, 51
Scheidel, Walter, 42–43
Science (journal), 25
secondary infection, defined, 30
septicemic plague (septicemia), 27
sexually transmitted infections (STIs), 24
smallpox
  deaths from, 34
  eradication of, 6
  fashion and, 39
  in research laboratories, 53
  spread of, 50
Snowden, Frank M.
  appearance of corpses of cholera victims, 25
  cholera symptoms, 24–25
  Middle Ages clothing to protect against plague, 14–15
  plague and establishment of public health systems, 44
  smallpox, 34
  symptoms of septicemic plague, 27
social norms, 40–42, **43**
socioeconomic status, 14
South Africa, 17, **20**
Spanish flu. *See* 1918 influenza (Spanish flu)
Spinney, Laura, 29–30
spread
  methods of, 10–11, 19–20, 50, **50**
  reproductive number and, 12
swine flu (H1N1 flu), 17

Taylor, Steven, 40
ticks, 53–54
tuberculosis (TB), **23**
  cause, 8
  deaths from, 22–23
  fashion and, 39

  HIV-positive people with, 22
  spread of, 10

United Nations Environment Programme (UNEP), 52

vaccines
  COVID-19, 35, 51
  MMR, 11
  operation of, 11
vectors, 11
viruses, 9

Wagner, Abram L., 10
Walsh, Kieran, 52
Wang, Jessica, 21
Washington Post (newspaper), 4
"waves" of infection, 10
World Bank, 50
World Economic Forum, 47–48
World Health Organization (WHO)
  antibiotic resistance, 48
  deaths from tuberculosis, 22
  diagnosis of HIV, 19
  Ebola fatality rate, 32
  Ebola outbreak in DRC (2020), 13, 32
  emergence of infectious diseases since 1970s, 6
  HIV-positive people with tuberculosis, 22
  major leading causes of death worldwide, 46
  malaria as endemic, 21
  malaria deaths, 21
  1918 influenza (Spanish flu), 31
  prevalence and deaths from cholera, 25
  prevalence of plague, 29
  prevalence of STIs, 24
  rabies, 21
  treatment of HIV, 19
Wuhan, China, 4
Wynes, Allison, 4

xenophobia, 38–40

Yong, Ed, 34

Zika virus, 13
zoonotic diseases, 51–52

PICTURE CREDITS

Cover: plrang/Depositphotos

 5: lev radin/Shutterstock.com
 9: Everett Collection/Shutterstock.com
12: fotohay/Shutterstock.com
15: Channarong Pherngjanda/Shutterstock.com
20: Associated Press
23: Pewadol Jaturawutthichai/Shutterstock.com
28: Associated Press
30: Everett Collection/Shutterstock.com
33: Alexandros Michailidis/Shutterstock.com
37: myboys.me/Shutterstock.com
43: YES Market Media/Shutterstock.com
49: pixelheadphoto digitalskillet/Shutterstock.com
50: pio3/Shutterstock.com

ABOUT THE AUTHOR

Andrea C. Nakaya, a native of New Zealand, holds a bachelor's degree in English and a master's degree in communications from San Diego State University. She has written and edited numerous articles, and more than fifty books, on current issues. She currently lives in Eagle, Idaho, with her husband and their two children, Natalie and Shane.